Happy Days with the Naked Chef

Jamie Oliver

ACCOMPANYING A MAJOR BBC TV SERIES

Happy Days with the Naked Chef

Jamie Oliver

with photographs by David Loftus

PENGUIN BOOKS

PENGUIN BOOKS

UK | USA | Canada | Ireland | Australia
India | New Zealand | South Africa

Penguin Books is part of the Penguin Random House group of companies
whose addresses can be found at global.penguinrandomhouse.com

First published by Michael Joseph 2001
Published in Penguin Books 2003
Reissued in this edition 2019
001

Printed in China

A CIP catalogue record for this book is available from the British Library

ISBN: 978–1–405–93353–7

penguin.co.uk

jamieoliver.com

www.greenpenguin.co.uk

Penguin Random House is committed to a
sustainable future for our business, our readers
and our planet. This book is made from Forest
Stewardship Council® certified paper.

CONTENTS

Dedicated to my brand new nephews Little Henners and Jakey Bakey

Gordon Bennett

– last year was busy but this one has been doolally! I'm in Cornwall writing this introduction, while being clicked at by photographers in bushes. Before you think it, I'm not getting tired of cooking. I think I'm even more obsessed! It's become a weekly occurrence to wake up after being bashed by my missus telling me that I've been muttering in my sleep about sweet red onions and fields of herbs – don't remember it, but it wouldn't surprise me. It didn't stop her marrying me – yep, Mr and Mrs Oliver we are now – and I think she still likes me!

On the big day itself we were up at 5 am cooking with my dad, Gennaro my London 'dad', my best man Bender the Aussie, and my chef mates from Monte's. What a fantastic day. All I wanted to see was our best friends and family really tucking in and having a laugh, so for starters I had lots of different tapas and antipasti, fresh bread and big plates of Parma ham, bresaola and salamis from Italy. Little bowls of chutneys and sauces went with them and it worked. Everyone was tucking in, passing stuff around, and from the top table it was a fantastic sight – definitely the feast of the year. For the main course we had whole wild salmon stuffed with loadsa herbs and baked with a little white wine and olive oil. This was served with lemon and basil mayonnaise, boiled potatoes dug up from Dad's garden that morning, and nice green salad. For dessert, the sweetest strawberries and some mascarpone cream. Lovely. So simple but perfect for a summer wedding.

Jools and my mum still act as a fantastic grounding for my cooking. After nine years of Jools hating everything about cooking I realized recently that I was being too honest about her attempts – no matter how I put it, she considered it a bit of a knockback, so I lied and said 'It's fantastic, babe!' to whatever she cooked for me. Since then she hasn't stopped cooking and has naturally got better and better. She now doesn't mind discussing the finer details and she's doing loadsa cooking at home. Everyone likes to feel that they're good at something and cooking is no exception. I do find Jools' opinion massively helpful in writing a book which must be accessible to everyone because if she can do it, so can you. What I've really enjoyed recently is cooking together – before, she used to heckle me from the stairs, which really used to wind me up. Now we're quite a good team in the kitchen and it means we get things done quicker.

Over the last year or so, I've done quite a bit of travelling which has been very inspiring on the old food front – Australia, New Zealand, America and Japan. Every country blew me away with a handful of genius dinners. There was the odd shocker, one of which came in the form of a bullock's bollocks in the US. And cod semen (disguised as chicken) in Japan – it's a delicacy over there and I was the guest of honour so I got the biggest portion. It tasted all right, but it just felt wrong.

I finished off the year by taking over as consultant chef at Monte's in Sloane Street, London. It has been a real challenge and education to launch a restaurant from scratch, following in the footsteps of chef Alain Ducasse, and I'm really happy with the young team that works for me in the kitchen, headed up by Bender the Aussie. And apart from that, we're busy. It's been great to carry on writing seasonal menus using the best produce while still searching for the perfect restaurant site of my own.

People keep asking me if the success of the books and the programmes has changed me and all my thoughts about food. Well, I think as a person I haven't really changed apart from having to grow up a bit. But from the feedback I've had in letters and e-mails to my website (jamieoliver.com) I definitely think I've got more of an idea about what the average person wants to cook at home. I've written *Happy Days* with this in mind.

I feel like this book has moved naturally on from the first two as it's still focusing on reality: being able to buy the best ingredients you can. You know what I mean, simple, comforting, homely food is still what it's all about. Foodwise, this year has been very creative for me and, as you'll see in the book, I've come up with loads of new recipes, as well as some really cool new chapters that I'm very excited about. The most important one is Kids' Club, which is all about getting parents to capture their kids' imaginations to get them involved and interested in food. Then there's Quick Fixes, which is all about quick, tasty dinners – ideal for when you get in late after a hard day's work. Comfort Grub is all your old favourites and some new ideas – to be eaten while snuggled up in front of the TV.

I'm really proud of *Happy Days* – to me it feels more like a diary than a cookbook, as it's my memories of the last couple of years and because of that it's very eclectic, with little fusions and ideas from my travels. I've included some classic recipes as well as putting a twist on others to reflect my personal taste. But, hey, that's what it's all about.

Cooking … happy days! Love Jamie. x

Cupboard Stuff

HERBS The question is why is a 26-year-old full-blooded Essex boy devoting two precious pages of his beloved book to herbs? I respect the fact that my lovely missus thinks I'm crackers with my obsession for the fragrant leaves, but quite frankly they're cool – not just cool, but very cool. If there were no herbs in this world I would give up cooking tomorrow; how boring would cooking be? With herbs you can completely transform a dish, make it heartier, lighter or more fragrant, and marry together all sorts of dishes that may never have worked without them. To grow them and have them right there at the kitchen window at their freshest is a cook's dream; to run out to get herbs to bash up in a pestle and mortar and rub over a nice piece of lamb with a little oil is the best.

If you're a real connoisseur of herbs you'll probably meet my mate Jekka along the way, be it at Chelsea Flower Show or at a festival. She's amazing, completely potty about herbs, nurturing and growing the most fantastic herb cuttings and seeds from all over the world, with looks, tastes and smells that you've never experienced before. It's like heaven to me; I'm already planning my herb garden in my non-existent garden. I've only known her for a short amount of time but that's the great thing about food or any passion really, it will always bring people together to become buddies.

All this little chapter is about is to say please try getting into herbs, they are a real trick to kick-starting your cooking. Not only that, but after a good gossip with Jekka, I was really shocked to find out that using herbs simply for flavouring is quite a new thing in the history of food. Different herbs were used as natural and accessible antiseptics that would aid digestion; herbs like sage can arrest the ageing process and can be found in some face creams, but originally sage was packed with meat to make it keep for much longer. Fennel, coriander, tarragon and dill are great for digestion and help break down cholesterol. Good old mint is an anti-inflammatory and stimulates the appetite. And rosemary is great for the liver and a great calming and stress-relieving herb. This is naming just a few, but the point is that even when you don't know it you're doing yourself a great deal of good when you use herbs in your cooking, so get stuck in and get out ya herbs.

COMFORT GRUB The idea of this chapter is to touch on a couple of those hearty, homely comfort grub dinners, like toad in the hole and a nice beef stew with 'Newkie Brown' ale and dumplings – meals for those lazy nights where you curl up in front of the telly and just chill out.

Comfort food can come from many countries with things like the ultimate chilli con carne, or the fluffiest American pancakes. With this chapter I wanted to reassure you that even though I'm a chef, I still get cravings for a good old fish finger buttie or sticky sausage & cheese bap with brown sauce. The one thing all these recipes have in common is normally memories of childhood; enjoying company round the dinner table, or in my case, coming home shivering and wet from playing footie with the boys and being ordered to change out of my wet clothes into my dressing gown before being given a steaming bowl of chilli with a jacket potato and a lob of guacamole and yoghurt. Remember: Don't eat to live, but live to eat. That's what it's all about!

Toad in the Hole

SERVES 4

sunflower oil • 8 quality sausages • 4 sprigs of fresh
rosemary • 2 large red onions, peeled and sliced •
2 cloves of garlic, peeled and finely sliced • 2 knobs of unsalted
butter • 6 tablespoons balsamic vinegar • 1 level tablespoon
vegetable stock powder or 1 vegetable stock cube

BATTER

300ml milk • 100g plain flour • 3 large eggs

Mix the batter ingredients together with a pinch of sea salt, and put to one side. I like the batter to go huge, so the key thing is to have an appropriately-sized baking tin – the thinner the better – as we need to get the oil smoking hot.

Put 2 tablespoons of oil into a baking tin, then place this on the middle shelf of the oven at full whack (240°C/475°F/gas 9). Place a larger tray underneath to catch any oil that overflows while cooking. When the oil is very hot, add the sausages. Keep an eye on them and allow them to colour until lightly golden.

At this point, take the tin out of the oven, being very careful, and pour the batter over the sausages. Throw a couple of sprigs of rosemary into the batter. It will bubble and possibly even spit a little, so put the tin back in the oven carefully, and close the door. Don't open it for at least 20 minutes, as Yorkshire puddings can be a bit temperamental when rising. Remove from the oven when golden and crisp.

For the onion gravy, simply fry the onions and garlic in the butter on a medium heat for about 5 minutes, or until sweet and translucent. You could add a little thyme or rosemary, if you like. Add the balsamic vinegar and allow it to cook down by half. At this point, I do cheat a little and add a stock cube or powder. You can get some good ones in the supermarkets now that aren't full of rubbish. Sprinkle this in and add a little water. Allow to simmer and you'll have a really tasty onion gravy. Take to the table with the toad in the hole – delicious served with mashed potatoes, greens and baked beans or maybe a green salad if you're feeling a little guilty!

CALORIES	FAT	SAT FAT	PROTEIN	CARBS	SUGAR	SALT	FIBRE
656kcal	44.3g	17.3g	27.4g	41.2g	17.7g	2.3g	3.6g

Good Old Steak & Guinness Pie

This is nice and easy to make as all you have to do is put a puff pastry lid on top of a dish filled with stewed meat. I never serve anything else with these pies, but if you want to, boiled potatoes and steamed greens always hit the spot.

SERVES 6

700g stewing beef, diced • 2 heaped tablespoons plain flour • olive oil • 1 onion, peeled and roughly chopped • 1 large carrot, peeled and roughly chopped • 4 sticks of celery, roughly chopped • 2 parsnips, peeled and roughly chopped • 1 bunch of fresh mixed herbs, such as rosemary, thyme, bay, leaves picked • 1 pint of Guinness • 2 x 400g tins of quality plum tomatoes • 1 x 500g pack of puff pastry • 1 large egg, beaten

Season the beef generously with sea salt and black pepper, sprinkle with the flour and toss to coat. Heat 2 or 3 lugs of oil in a large casserole pan and fry the meat in 2 batches until golden brown. Add the onion and fry for 1 more minute, then add the carrot, celery, parsnips and herbs. Fry for a further 4 minutes, then pour in the Guinness. Add the tomatoes, breaking them up with a wooden spoon, and bring to the boil. Stir well, then simmer for 2 hours, or until really tender – the sauce should be nice and thick with an intensely tasty flavour. Season with salt and pepper. At this point you could serve it as a stew with mash, or it will keep really well for a good 3 days in the fridge (while improving in flavour at the same time).

To make the pies, preheat the oven to 190°C/375°F/gas 5. Put the meat filling into an appropriately-sized baking dish or dishes. I like to make small individual pies – any high-sided round ovenproof bowls are fine. Roll out the pastry, dusting with flour as you go, until ½cm thick. Cut out 6 circles about 1cm bigger than the tops of the bowls. Brush the rims of the bowls with beaten egg, then place the pastry circles on top, squashing the excess pastry down the outside of the bowls to secure. Lightly score the top of the pastry in a criss-cross fashion and brush with more beaten egg. Bake in the middle of the oven for 45 minutes, or until golden.

CALORIES	FAT	SAT FAT	PROTEIN	CARBS	SUGAR	SALT	FIBRE
689kcal	37g	14.6g	34.4g	52.4g	15.8g	1.2g	7.4g

Beef Stew with Newcastle Brown Ale & Dumplings

SERVES 6–8

1kg shin of beef (or use flank or neck), chopped into chunks •
3 tablespoons plain flour • olive oil • 3 red onions, peeled
and roughly sliced • 50g pancetta or smoked streaky bacon,
chopped • 3 sticks of celery, chopped • ½ a bunch of fresh
rosemary, leaves picked • 2 pints of Newcastle Brown ale •
2 parsnips, peeled and roughly chopped • 2 carrots, peeled and
roughly chopped • 4 potatoes, peeled and roughly chopped

DUMPLINGS

225g self-raising flour • 115g unsalted butter • 2 sprigs of fresh
rosemary, picked and chopped

Season the beef with sea salt and black pepper, sprinkle with the flour and toss around until well coated. Heat up a frying pan until it is good and hot, add a little oil and fry the beef in 2 batches until golden brown. Transfer the meat to a big casserole – one which is suitable to go on a hob – mixing in the flour that was left on the plate after coating it. Put the casserole on a medium heat, add the onions and pancetta, and cook until the onions are translucent and the pancetta has a bit of colour. Add the celery and rosemary. Pour in the Newcastle Brown ale and 300ml of water, then add the parsnips, carrots and potatoes (feel free to add whatever veg you like at this stage). Bring to the boil, put a lid on, turn down the heat and leave to simmer while you make the dumplings – which are choice.

Blitz the dumpling ingredients in a blender or rub between your fingers till you have a breadcrumb consistency, then add just enough water to make a dough that isn't sticky. Divide it into ping-pong-ball sized dumplings and put these into the stew, dunking them under. Put the lid back on and leave it to cook for 2 hours. Taste it, season it as you like, then serve with some cavolo nero or other greens and loads of bread to mop up the juices, if you like.

CALORIES	FAT	SAT FAT	PROTEIN	CARBS	SUGAR	SALT	FIBRE
684kcal	37g	14.6g	33.6g	52.4g	15.8g	1.2g	7.6g

Chilli con Carne

It's great to buy chuck steak for this recipe because you know exactly what quality of meat you're buying. Simply cut it into pieces and pulse in a food processor until it resembles minced beef. I normally make double the amount of chilli needed so that I can divide the extra into sandwich bags, knotted at the top, for freezing. These bags can then be boiled for 15 minutes when needed.

SERVES 4

2 medium onions • 1 clove of garlic • olive oil • 2 level teaspoons chilli powder • 1 fresh red chilli, deseeded and finely chopped • 1 heaped teaspoon ground cumin (or crushed cumin seeds) • 450g chuck steak, minced, or quality minced beef • 200g sun-dried tomatoes, in oil • 2 x 400g tins of quality plum tomatoes • ½ a stick of cinnamon • 2 x 400g tins of red kidney beans, drained

To cook this I use a metal pan or casserole with a lid, which you can use on the hob and in the oven. If you are going to use the oven method (see below), preheat the oven to 150°C/300°F/gas 2. Blitz the onions and garlic in a food processor until finely chopped, then fry in a little olive oil until soft. Add the chilli powder, fresh chilli, cumin and a little sea salt and black pepper. Add the minced chuck steak or beef and continue to cook, stirring, until golden brown. Blitz the sun-dried tomatoes in the food processor with enough oil from the jar to loosen into a paste. Add this to the beef with the tomatoes, cinnamon and a wineglass of water. Season a little more with salt and pepper, if needed.

Bring to the boil, cover with greaseproof paper and the lid, then either turn the heat down to simmer and cook for 1 hour 30 minutes, or transfer the pan to the oven for 1 hour 30 minutes. Add the tinned kidney beans 30 minutes before the end of the cooking time – they're already cooked and only need warming up.

This always tastes better if you cook it the day before (to give the flavours time to develop), so it's really handy if you've got friends coming round and don't want to be stuck in the kitchen. Just take it out of the fridge and warm it up – delicious served with fresh crusty bread, green salad and natural yoghurt or guacamole.

CALORIES	FAT	SAT FAT	PROTEIN	CARBS	SUGAR	SALT	FIBRE
460kcal	12.1g	2.5g	41.3g	49.2g	21.2g	3.5g	7.5g

My Favourite Curry Sauce

You will really like this curry – it's easy and fun to make. Two little tips – first, use a food processor to chop the onions and tomatoes as it makes less mess, it's really quick and will stop you crying! Second, get all the ingredients prepped and ready to go, then you can have the sauce finished in just 15 minutes. Keep your eyes peeled for curry leaves – I'm trying to get supermarkets to stock them at the moment, but you can buy them from Indian or Asian delis. Buy a big bag, let them dry and they'll last for ages. If you really can't get them, do without, but it won't be quite the same.

SERVES 4

vegetable oil • 2 teaspoons mustard seeds • 1 teaspoon fenugreek seeds • 3 fresh green chillies, deseeded and finely sliced • 1 handful of curry leaves • 10cm piece of ginger, peeled and coarsely grated • 3 onions, peeled and chopped • 1 teaspoon chilli powder • 1 teaspoon ground turmeric • 6 ripe tomatoes, chopped • 1 x 400ml tin of light coconut milk

CALORIES	FAT	SAT FAT	PROTEIN	CARBS	SUGAR	SALT	FIBRE
293kcal	24g	6.5g	4.4g	18.2g	14.8g	0.5g	5.2g

FISH VERSION

4 x 225g haddock fillets, skin off, pin-boned • 1 knob of tamarind paste or 1 teaspoon tamarind syrup • optional: 1 large handful of baby spinach • optional: 1 bunch of fresh coriander, picked and chopped

CHICKEN VERSION

4 chicken breasts, sliced into 1cm strips • 1 tablespoon coriander seeds, crushed

VEGETARIAN VERSION

800g mixed vegetables, such as potatoes, courgettes, peppers, onions, sweet potatoes, spinach, chard, cauliflower, lentils, beans, prepped and chopped

Heat 5 tablespoons of oil in a pan, and when hot add the mustard seeds. Wait for them to pop, then add the fenugreek seeds, fresh green chillies, curry leaves and ginger. Stir and fry for a few minutes. Use a food processor to chop the onions and add to the pan. Continue to cook for 5 minutes, or until the onions are soft, then add the chilli powder and turmeric. Pulse the tomatoes in the food processor and add to the pan. Cook for a couple of minutes, then pour in 1 or 2 wineglasses of water and the coconut milk. Simmer for 5 minutes, or until it has the consistency of double cream, then season carefully with sea salt.

Use this sauce as a base. To make the fish curry, add the fish and tamarind to the sauce and simmer for 6 minutes. Feel free to add some baby spinach and chopped coriander at the end of the cooking time. For the chicken version, stir-fry the chicken strips and coriander seeds until golden, then add to the sauce and simmer for 10 minutes, or until cooked through. For the vegetarian version, simply add all the veg to the sauce at the beginning when you add the onions. Continue to cook as normal and simmer until just tender.

Lemon Rice

I've always wanted to know how Indian and Thai chefs make tasty rice. This is a great way to liven up plain rice, but feel free to take it a step further by adding ground turmeric, like my Indian friend Das. Or hot it up with a little chilli powder. You can also toast some broken unsalted nuts, scramble in some eggs, or try any ideas or flavour combinations that you think are delicious.

SERVES 6

450g basmati rice • vegetable oil • 2 tablespoons mustard
seeds • 2 teaspoons urad dhal (small dried split peas) •
1 handful of curry leaves • 2 lemons • 1 bunch of fresh
coriander, leaves picked and chopped

Throw the rice into boiling water, cook for 10 minutes and drain.

Heat 5 tablespoons of oil in a small frying pan over a medium heat. Add the mustard seeds and as they begin to pop add the urad dhal, curry leaves and strips of lemon rind (remove these with a vegetable peeler). Leave to cook for 1 minute, or until the urad dhal and lemon peel are lightly coloured.

Put the drained steaming rice into a bowl and pour over the cooked spices. Squeeze over the lemon juice and stir through the chopped coriander. Season to taste with sea salt and black pepper. Delicious served with curry (see page 32).

CALORIES	FAT	SAT FAT	PROTEIN	CARBS	SUGAR	SALT	FIBRE
377kcal	11.8g	1.3g	6.7g	61.5g	0.3g	0.3g	0g

Coriander Chutney

400g natural yoghurt • 1 bunch of fresh coriander, leaves picked • 2–3 cloves of garlic • 2.5cm piece of ginger • 2 green chillies, seeds removed • juice of ½ a lime

Place all the ingredients in a food processor with a pinch of sea salt and blend until smooth. This will keep in the fridge for 3 days.

CALORIES	FAT	SAT FAT	PROTEIN	CARBS	SUGAR	SALT	FIBRE
15kcal	0.7g	0.5g	0.9g	1.2g	1.1g	0.1g	0g

THESE VALUES ARE BASED ON 1 TABLESPOON

Lemon Pickle

2 teaspoons mustard seeds • olive oil • optional: 1 small handful
of curry leaves • optional: 1 teaspoon urad dhal (small dried split
peas) • 1 teaspoon chilli powder • 4 tablespoons wine vinegar
• 2 lemons, deseeded and chopped

Fry the mustard seeds in 2 tablespoons of hot oil. As they begin to pop add the
curry leaves and urad dhal. Lower the heat and add the chilli powder; cook until
brown, then add the vinegar. Stir in the lemon, remove from the heat and leave
to cool. This will keep in the fridge for 3 days.

CALORIES	FAT	SAT FAT	PROTEIN	CARBS	SUGAR	SALT	FIBRE
21kcal	2.2g	0.3g	0.4g	0.4g	0.4g	0g	0.1g

THESE VALUES ARE BASED ON 1 TABLESPOON

Fantastic Fish Finger Buttie

As a chef I always feel I shouldn't be eating something like a fish finger buttie – but you know what, I think that makes it taste even better. Here's what I do . . .

I remove about 4 fish fingers from the freezer and grill them on each side until crispy and golden. While that's happening, I butter 2 bits of nice soft white bread or a white roll, spreading one half generously with tomato ketchup. When the fish fingers are done, I remove them from the grill and place them on the bread covered with ketchup. The most important bit is to put the other bit of bread on top and, using a little force, push down on your buttie which, for some reason, seems to make it taste even better. And that's it – all done.

I tend to eat one of these while I'm walking about at home and I always get told off by the missus for dropping bits everywhere. You'll notice from the picture that I've put a handful of rocket in the sandwich, which isn't really necessary but it does make it look a bit more posh. I was a bit embarrassed to tell the photographer he had to shoot a fish finger sandwich, so I told him it was 'lemon sole goujons' – what a prat I am! Be proud to eat fish fingers, that's what I say.

CALORIES	FAT	SAT FAT	PROTEIN	CARBS	SUGAR	SALT	FIBRE
461kcal	18.5g	7.7g	19.7g	57.7g	6.2g	3g	1.9g

Sticky Sausage Bap
with Melted Cheese & Brown Sauce

I used to have one of these every morning at 7 am on the way to college at Westminster. Just get 3 half-decent snags (that's sausages to us southerners) and grill them until sticky and crispy on all sides. Remove to a plate, cut them in half, and line them up in the grill tray in the shape of your bap. Cover evenly with a good handful of grated mild Cheddar cheese and put back under the grill for the cheese to melt. Slice your bap in half, butter both sides, and smear outrageously with brown sauce. Using a knife, place your sausages and melted cheese on the brown sauce side of the bap. Then push the other side down on top of it and tuck in!

CALORIES	FAT	SAT FAT	PROTEIN	CARBS	SUGAR	SALT	FIBRE
654kcal	38.2g	16.6g	35.1g	44.5g	7g	3.1g	2.6g

Pancakes USA Stylie

These American pancakes are great! Instead of being thin and silky like French crêpes, they are wonderfully fluffy and thick and can be made to perfection straight away. Simple, simple, simple – my Jools goes mad for them!

SERVES 4

3 large eggs • 100g plain flour •
1 heaped teaspoon baking powder • 140ml milk

First separate the eggs, putting the whites into one bowl and the yolks into another. Add the flour, baking powder and milk to the yolks and mix to a smooth thick batter. Whisk the whites with a pinch of sea salt until they form stiff peaks. Fold into the batter – it's now ready to use.

Heat a non-stick pan over a medium heat. Pour some of the batter into the pan and fry for a couple of minutes, or until it starts to look golden and firm. At this point sprinkle your chosen flavouring (see below) on to the uncooked side before loosening with a spatula and quickly and confidently flipping the pancake over. Continue frying until both sides are beautifully golden.

You can make these pancakes large or small, to your liking. You can serve them simply doused in maple syrup and even with some butter or crème fraîche. Or if you choose to sprinkle with a flavouring, try one of these . . .

fresh corn (see page 41) • crispy smoked bacon or
pancetta • blueberries • banana • stewed apple •
grated chocolate • anything else you can imagine . . .

CALORIES	FAT	SAT FAT	PROTEIN	CARBS	SUGAR	SALT	FIBRE
167kcal	5.7g	1.7g	9g	21.8g	2.2g	1.2g	0.8g

PS Blueberry pancakes (above) are great but you must try the corn pancakes. On one condition – you must use fresh corn. To do this, remove the outer leaves and carefully run a knife down the cob – this will loosen all the lovely pieces of corn – and sprinkle these raw over your pancake, before flipping it in the pan. I like to have some grilled bacon over my corn pancakes, drizzled with a little maple syrup. This sounds bloody horrid but it honestly tastes pukka!

QUICK FIXES This chapter is all about really fast tasty ways to eat good old chicken, steak, cod and salmon, time and minimal washing up being of the essence. I'm going to give you quick methods like frying or grilling, or my favourite, baking in the bag, which I started doing when Jools and I first moved to London six years ago – with me having been briefed by the lovely mother-in-law to 'look after my little baby'. We were completely skint, our kitchen was the size of an airing-cupboard and we were working opposite shifts to each other. I didn't want Jools to feed herself on ready meals so I found myself custom-making the fantastic 'Jamie Oliver dinners in a bag', involving the glorious tin foil. I've got a thing about tin foil – people must think either I'm a bit kinky because I use so much of it, or that I sponsor NASA!

I love making these little envelopes, or bags, with all the ingredients placed in the middle of them. What this means is that there's no washing up (just tin foil in the bin), you don't have to use that much fat, just a little olive oil will do, and you can do pretty much any combination you like. But the great thing is that you cook your meat or fish in the same bag as the vegetables and herbs, which, in return, gives you a healthy, homemade sauce which is great. The two baking-in-the-bag recipes I'm going to give you here use chicken, but you can do all kinds of fish, noodles, or a vegetarian bag.

What I would do for Jools was make up a combo at 4 pm, as I was going off to work, and write with a marker pen '20 minutes at 200ºC', for example, on the foil. Even though Jools didn't like cooking, she never had a problem with cooking the bags.

Chicken Baked in a Bag
with Mushrooms, Butter, White Wine & Thyme

SERVES 2

2 x 200g skinless chicken breasts • 1 handful of dried porcini mushrooms • 250g mixed mushrooms, torn up • 1 large wineglass of white wine • 3 large knobs of unsalted butter • 1 handful of fresh thyme • 2 cloves of garlic, peeled and sliced

As this is for 2 people, I'm going to make a large envelope/bag to cook everything in. Using wide tin foil, make the bag by placing 2 pieces on top of each other (about as big as 2 shoeboxes in length), folding 3 sides in and leaving 1 side open.

Preheat the oven to 220°C/425°F/gas 7. Mix everything together in a bowl, including the chicken. Place in the bag, with all the liquid, making sure you don't pierce the foil. Close up the final edge, making sure the bag is tightly sealed and secure on all sides, and carefully slide it on to a roasting tray. Place the tray on a high heat on the hob for 1 minute to get the heat going, then bake in the middle of the oven for 25 minutes.

Remove from the oven, place the bag on a big plate, take it to the table and carefully break open the foil. Feel free to vary the recipe – things like grated parsnip, smoked bacon and red wine also work well.

CALORIES	FAT	SAT FAT	PROTEIN	CARBS	SUGAR	SALT	FIBRE
421kcal	15g	8.5g	51.5g	4.3g	1.4g	0.3g	2.4g

Chicken Baked in a Bag
with Cannellini Beans, Leeks, Cream & Marjoram

10 baby leeks, trimmed and washed • 2 x 200g skinless chicken breasts • 1 x 400g tin of cannellini beans, drained and washed • 1 clove of garlic, peeled and sliced • ½ a bunch of fresh marjoram or oregano, leaves picked • 1 small wineglass of white wine • 100ml double cream

As this is for 2 people, I'm going to make a large envelope/bag to cook everything in. Using wide tin foil, make the bag by placing 2 pieces on top of each other (about as big as 2 shoeboxes in length), folding 3 sides in and leaving 1 side open.

Preheat the oven to 220°C/425°F/gas 7. Put the leeks into a pan and cook in boiling water for 2 minutes, just to soften. Drain and mix in a bowl with all the other ingredients, including the chicken, mushing a handful of the cannellini beans to a pulp in your hands. Season well with sea salt and black pepper, then place in the bag with all the creamy sauce, making sure you don't pierce the foil. Close up the final edge, making sure the bag is tightly sealed and secure on all sides, and carefully slide it on to a roasting tray. Place the tray on a high heat on the hob for 1 minute to get the heat going, then bake in the middle of the oven for 25 minutes.

Remove from the oven, place the bag on a big plate, take it to the table and carefully break open the foil. Feel free to vary the recipe – things like cooked new potatoes, a little wholegrain mustard or baby spinach are all good.

CALORIES	FAT	SAT FAT	PROTEIN	CARBS	SUGAR	SALT	FIBRE
647kcal	30.9g	17.6g	58.9g	18.3g	4.3g	0.9g	11g

Sirloin of Beef
with Pak Choi, Soy Sauce & Ginger

SERVES 2

2 x 200g sirloin steaks • 2 pak choi or bok choi (even spinach
or any other greens will do) • 8 tablespoons low-salt soy
sauce • ½ a clove of garlic, finely grated • 5cm piece of ginger,
peeled and finely grated • 1 fresh red chilli, deseeded and finely
grated • extra virgin olive oil • 1 lime

Season the steaks on both sides with black pepper. On a very hot griddle, cook
the steaks until medium or to your liking. Place on a plate and allow to rest for
2 minutes, then cook your greens in boiling salted water until tender. While hot,
douse the steaks with the soy sauce, and sprinkle with the garlic, ginger and chilli.
Drizzle with 2 tablespoons of oil and squeeze over the lime juice. When the greens
are cooked, simply divide between 2 plates, slice up the steaks, place on top of the
greens and drizzle with any of the infused sauce left on the resting plate.

CALORIES	FAT	SAT FAT	PROTEIN	CARBS	SUGAR	SALT	FIBRE
435kcal	28.5g	8.9g	36.6g	8.1g	4g	4.7g	2.2g

The Best Steak Sarnie

SERVES 2

1 ciabatta loaf or baguette • 1 x 300g rump steak •
2 sprigs of fresh rosemary, leaves picked • olive oil •
1 lemon • extra virgin olive oil • 1–2 tablespoons Dijon
mustard • 1 handful of rocket or watercress

Place the ciabatta in the oven to warm for a few minutes at 100ºC/225ºF/gas ¼. Season the steak with sea salt and black pepper, then sprinkle it with rosemary. Slice it across in half, place the slices one at a time between 2 pieces of clingfilm, and bash with a flat heavy object like a pot or cleaver or even your fist until 1cm thick. Rub with a little olive oil, place on a very hot griddle or frying pan and sear for 1 minute on each side. This will cook the meat pink, but you can cook it less or more to your liking. Remove to a plate, squeeze over the lemon juice and allow to rest while you cut the ciabatta in half lengthways and drizzle the cut sides with extra virgin olive oil. Spread a dollop of Dijon mustard over the bread, put the steak and rocket on top, then drizzle over any resting juices. Squeeze together and eat!

CALORIES	FAT	SAT FAT	PROTEIN	CARBS	SUGAR	SALT	FIBRE
568kcal	14.8g	3.7g	42.4g	70.6g	4.2g	2.3g	5g

Baked Cod
with Avocado, Prawns, Cream & Cheese

SERVES 2

olive oil • 2 x 225g cod fillets, skin off, pin-boned • 1 small
handful of fresh basil, ripped • ½ an avocado, peeled, stoned,
and sliced • 150g large peeled prawns, cooked or uncooked
• 65ml double cream • 65g mature Cheddar cheese

Preheat the oven to 220°C/425°F/gas 7. Rub a baking dish or roasting tray with
a little oil, season the cod on both sides with sea salt and black pepper and place
in the dish. Sprinkle the fillets with the basil, avocado and prawns. Drizzle over the
cream and grate over the cheese. Cook at the top of the oven for 15 to 20 minutes,
or until golden and bubbling. Serve simply with a green salad. Lovely jubbly.

CALORIES	FAT	SAT FAT	PROTEIN	CARBS	SUGAR	SALT	FIBRE
852kcal	62.9g	35.1g	69.6g	2g	1.2g	2.6g	0.1g

Roasted Cod
with Cherry Tomatoes, Basil & Mozzarella

SERVES 2

2 x 225g cod fillets, skin off, pin-boned • olive oil • 2 handfuls
of red and yellow cherry tomatoes, halved • 1 bunch of fresh
basil, leaves picked • 1 ball of buffalo mozzarella cheese, finely
sliced • 1 handful of freshly grated Parmesan cheese

Preheat the oven to 220°C/425°F/gas 7. Place the cod fillets in an oiled roasting tray or an earthenware dish. Drizzle with oil and season with sea salt and black pepper. Place the tomatoes, basil and mozzarella on top of the fillets. Sprinkle over the Parmesan, drizzle over some oil, and bake at the top of the oven for 15 to 20 minutes, or until golden. Serve simply with a green salad. Delicious!

CALORIES	FAT	SAT FAT	PROTEIN	CARBS	SUGAR	SALT	FIBRE
430kcal	20.9g	12.2g	57.6g	3.4g	3.1g	1.9g	1.2g

Seared Salmon
with Radicchio, Pancetta, Pine Nuts & Balsamic Vinegar

SERVES 2

1 radicchio, halved through the core and sliced • 8 rashers
of pancetta or dry-cured smoked streaky bacon • 1 bunch of
fresh marjoram or basil, leaves picked • 1 handful of pine nuts,
toasted • extra virgin olive oil • balsamic vinegar •
2 x 225g salmon fillets, skin off, pin-boned

Place the slices of radicchio on a very hot griddle pan and char for 1 minute on each side. Remove to a bowl. Cook the pancetta or bacon on the griddle, then remove and add to the radicchio. Throw the marjoram and toasted pine nuts into the bowl and drizzle with 2 or 3 good lugs of extra virgin olive oil. Add 2 or 3 tablespoons of balsamic vinegar, toss gently to coat and season to taste with sea salt and black pepper. Sear the salmon until just pink in the middle and serve straight away with the radicchio and pancetta.

CALORIES	FAT	SAT FAT	PROTEIN	CARBS	SUGAR	SALT	FIBRE
745kcal	54g	10.1g	58.1g	6.4g	5.9g	1.8g	1.3g

Salmon with Horseradish & Beets

SERVES 2

2 x 225g salmon fillets, skin on, scaled, pin-boned, scored
½cm deep • 6–8 baby beetroots, cooked until tender, then
sliced • ½ a bunch of fresh marjoram, leaves picked • extra
virgin olive oil • balsamic vinegar • 2 tablespoons crème
fraîche • 2 tablespoons creamed horseradish • 1 lemon
• 1 handful of rocket or watercress

Put the salmon fillets, skin side down, into a hot non-stick frying pan. Lightly press with a spatula so they don't curl up. After 1 minute they should be lightly golden. Turn the salmon over, sprinkle with sea salt, then place under the grill for 10 to 15 minutes, or until just cooked. While cooking, marinate the beetroots with the marjoram, a little oil, balsamic vinegar, salt and black pepper. Mix the crème fraîche with the horseradish and season to taste, carefully, with salt, pepper and lemon juice. Place the beets and salmon on serving plates, sprinkle over the rocket and drizzle with the horseradish sauce.

CALORIES	FAT	SAT FAT	PROTEIN	CARBS	SUGAR	SALT	FIBRE
635kcal	40.9g	10.5g	52.8g	14.7g	13.6g	1.3g	2.8g

kids'

club

HAVING A LAUGH

The title of this chapter may suggest otherwise, but it's really for parents. Getting your kids involved with food is definitely the way forward for cooking in this country. Shopping for the best ingredients, then cooking and eating good-quality food with them, is so incredibly important. Get your kids interested in all aspects of food – as well as being lots of fun it can also be an education for them, which will stand them in good stead for later life. As I'm not a father (yet), this chapter is not inspired by being a father – it's much more about the kid I was when I first started cooking. About what caught my attention and fascinated me. Get your kids interested and, trust me, you'll be on to a winner!

I now have a few friends with kids who really swear by getting them involved in the kitchen – I feel very strongly that parents have a responsibility to educate their kids not only to enjoy good food and understand it, but to take an interest in what they eat. This part of the book isn't about giving you 10 or 15 recipes and saying, 'Oh, and by the way these are for kids' – I think that's the wrong attitude. I'd like to think that kids can certainly get involved in some way in every single recipe in this book – obviously things like hot caramel, pans and sharp knives are no-nos for your bambinos, but there will always be little jobs that they can help with or do.

Most importantly, cooking with your kids is not about making smiley faces on pizzas or baking hedgehog cookies and disguising food. It's about smelling, touching, creating, tasting, laughing and eating. I've got a handful of recipes in this chapter which are always a great laugh and success with the kids, but to be honest it's more about a vibe; capturing the attention and imagination of the young ones. I'd like to think it will encourage them to feel free to roam through the rest of the book, cooking anything they like with a little help from their parents.

THE TRADE-OFF

As always when it comes to kids, to begin with you will find yourself in a trade-off situation! When I was five, my mum, dad and all their chefs at the pub used to get me involved in cooking to keep me quiet for 20 minutes and to get some little jobs done. In return they would give me and my friends some ice cream or push me on the rope swing for half an hour until I was sick – there was always a trade-off between me and them. You will soon find that trade-offs such as 'If you help me pod these peas, I'll make that favourite dessert of yours,' or 'If you don't help me I'll make you watch that Naked Chef on the TV,' will work wonders!

EDUCATION

Without sounding like a goody-goody or a preacher, in general kids' diets in Britain are a nightmare. Supermarkets, school dinners and cookery lessons should all try to help give families more knowledge about food. Just look at 90 per cent of kids' menus in restaurants – they're all the same: fish fingers, burgers, chicken nuggets and sausages. I'm not saying it's a bad thing and I know a lot of parents say, 'It's the only thing my little Joey will eat,' but some of the best experiences in my life, not only those involving food, have come through being forced to do or try different things. On a trip to Italy I saw a family with several small kids all tucking into grilled pigeon and gnawing the meat off the bones. They were also dipping crispy polenta into a spicy tomato sauce and loving it! It's terrific to see kids tucking in and enjoying tasty food without being worried about its colour, shape or texture. But also it's up to parents to make eating these types of foods a really exciting event. Try bigging up the more adventurous things by saying things like, 'Oh, isn't that lovely! Aren't you lucky, that'll put hairs on your chest' (cliché, cliché!). Good body language around food and kids also does the trick; smiles and coos of delight will all work. My mum and dad would encourage my sister and me to try things like crab and lobster with them – I didn't want to miss out on anything, so I tucked in.

SHOPPING

When I was as little as five years old, my dad used to take me to the fruit and veg market and cash and carry to get the essentials. I honestly used to feel slightly more grown-up and completely honoured when Dad used to say, 'Go on, son, I want you to go and pick me the best box of raspberries. Make sure you taste them, all right', which I used to do with great concentration. He used to have me groping melons, eating apples and sniffing herbs. I would scurry back with my opinion and some for him to try. Then we'd negotiate a price together and put it all in the van to go back to the pub. Even though I loved it, I think my dad used to take liberties with me being too keen, as he would say, 'Listen to Dad and go and tell that man over there that his fruit and veg is too expensive and a load of old rubbish.' Which I did with great conviction – resulting in me legging it from the warehouse!

So really try to get the kids involved in making some shopping decisions, because all they want is to be treated like grown-ups. Instead of letting them trail behind you while you pile things into the trolley, ask them to choose a pineapple by smelling it to check that it's ripe, for instance. Kids are like sponges – they soak up information and remember everything – so talk to them, ask for their opinions on what fish looks good or what meat to try. This can be good fun, especially when you reach the deli counter, as you can try out different things with them. Ask your kids to taste things like Parma ham, then ask them what they think. No matter what, always let them have some input when out shopping and listen to them seriously. If they realize their opinion counts then they will want to get involved when it comes to cooking and eating the ingredients.

CAPTURING THEIR IMAGINATION

As a kid I wasn't really that passionate about food, so it wasn't like I was born to cook. But living in a pub I did get to see a lot of preparation and different types of cooking from a young age, which was handy. Kids can get involved in all sorts of ways when it comes to cooking. There's so much more to learn from food than just eating it. I couldn't believe my eyes when I saw a piece of dough doubled in size and looking like The Blob! It was alive and I was absolutely mesmerized. How mad was that – something doubling in size over forty minutes. I was completely fascinated by the whole process: the proving, the shaping, the flavouring.

A CRAVING FOR COOKING

I craved responsibility as a kid. I wanted jobs to do; I wanted to muck in with everyone else. These days, I don't think enough responsibility for cooking is given to kids — maybe because parents are worried about them making a mess. It's so easy though; just teach them to make a great salad dressing in a jam jar — they can handle doing that. Then get them making the whole salad. And thank them for it — they'll want to do more. Some parents say, 'I'm going to cook with the kids today,' and they just bake gingerbread men and stuff like that. This is great, but try to get them involved here and there all the time if you can. That's what it's all about. But remember, it's not about ramming it down their throats either, so find a balance to suit you. Kids should be able to make just about anything in this book, but watch out for things that involve excess heat, sharp knives and machinery, plastic bags and clingfilm, which is not the end of the world because there is still a load of bashing, smashing, squeezing, stirring, tossing, drizzling and whipping to be done.

Here are some cooking ideas to try out with your kids:

Make marinades and bash spices in a pestle and mortar • Bash olives on a chopping board to remove the stones using one of their favourite mugs, like Thomas the Tank Engine, or something heavy; the stones should then be dropped into the mug — as sounds are so important in the kitchen, explain to your child that they should listen out for the stone hitting the mug • Pour oil over meat, fish or salads from a height • Pick herbs from the garden, smell them and rip them over a salad or finished pasta dish • Squeeze lemons • Squash tomatoes • Spin or toss salad leaves • Watch bread dough prove and check on it • Mash veg • And so much more . . .

IT'S A FAMILY THING

When talking to adults who are passionate about food, you'll very often find that they'll reminisce about their mum in the kitchen. This shows how important parents are when we think of food. When I was growing up and we lived above the pub, we would have our dinner at half five every day. That was our time to sit down together as a family, which, looking back, was so important. It was a time for laughing and sharing. It's nice to get everyone around the table and turn the TV off (unless the World Cup is on, of course) and simply enjoy eating together.

Dried Fruitgums

A few of my friends feed their kids really nice dried apricots, plums, peaches, pineapple and apples as a treat instead of giving them boiled sugar sweets. Surprisingly the kids absolutely love them. I actually think that a little paper bag of dried fruit is quite cool, but my friends fool their bambinos by cutting the fruit into shapes to look more like sweets.

When I cook these 'fruitgums' I normally do about 500g or a kilo of dried fruit at a time. You can do single types of fruit, or combos like mango and pineapple or peach and apricot. I simply whiz the dried fruit down to a very smooth purée in a food processor, then scoop it out on to some greased greaseproof paper. Using a palette knife, spread it out into a square, about ½cm thick. Then slide this on to a baking tray. I normally heat the fruit purée in the electric oven at 70°C/150°F overnight, which is very convenient for me, or, if you're in a rush, heat it at 160°C/300°F/gas 2 for a couple of hours – the cooking time really depends on how ripe and juicy the fruit was to start with.

When it's done, your layer of fruit should be soft but firm, a little bit like a winegum. Remove it from the oven to a chopping board, peel off the greaseproof paper and slice the fruit into small bite-sized pieces. Make a variety of shapes – squares, triangles, circles, strips. These can be kept in an airtight jar until you need them. It's lovely to wrap a few in a little paper bag and put them in your kids' lunchboxes. They'll really love 'em.

CALORIES	FAT	SAT FAT	PROTEIN	CARBS	SUGAR	SALT	FIBRE
135kcal	0.4g	0g	1.8g	33.2g	33.2g	0.1g	4g

THESE VALUES ARE BASED ON A 30G SERVING

Lollipops

My lovely nan and grandad used to run a village pub called the Plough and Sail in Paglesham in Essex. When I was a kid they used to send me and my sister, Anna-Marie, a huge box of about 200 ice lollies at the start of the summer holidays every year. The ice lollies would arrive with the deliveries from the same butcher that we've always shared and we would keep them in the big chest freezer outside in the store shed. This was great, as it meant I had a constant supply I could help myself to. I was always quite popular with the local kids because of this. So much so that my supplies would dwindle very quickly. So, I started to make my own lollipops.

The nice thing about them was that they weren't full of a thousand artificial ingredients because I would make them out of apple, orange, and pineapple juice – all sorts of stuff. Even cocktail combinations are good. I would also sneak into the pub for some cider shandy to make lollipops!

All you need to do to make lollipops is buy a couple of those really cheap moulds. You can find them in most kitchen shops. Fill them up with your chosen juice and put the stick in before freezing. It's nice to have something cold and fruity to hand in your freezer when it's a scorcher outside.

CALORIES	FAT	SAT FAT	PROTEIN	CARBS	SUGAR	SALT	FIBRE
0kcal	0g	0.1g	6.1g	6.1g	0g	0g	1g

Smush Ins

Smush ins are one of the coolest things to make (see pages 62–3). I remember when I was a kid, me and my sister would always try to defrost our hard ice cream in our dessert bowls into almost a thick milkshakey consistency before scoffing the lot. Then as we matured we realized that many flavours could be mushed in to improve the rubbishy ice cream that our parents always used to buy.

So, from the word 'mush' and the phrase 'mushing it in' they became 'smushins'. It was great going round the supermarkets as a kid secretly slipping possible smush ins into the trolley. Anything could be a contender – from fruit to maple syrup to smashed chocolate, or meringue – you name it, we would smush it! Winegums aren't good though. But melted chocolate caramel bars are chooooooooice.

All you need to do is get a big pot of vanilla ice cream and a selection of possible smush ins (see the picture on the next page for inspiration). Take 2 scoops of ice cream per person, blob these on to a clean chopping board, sprinkle or drizzle over your flavours, then, with a spatula or fork, mush and smush them together. Scoop up and lob into a bowl or cornet.

Give these a bash and make an event of them when you've got all the kids round. They're really good fun and great to use as bribes to get the kids helping you with the proper cooking! Smush away.

CALORIES	FAT	SAT FAT	PROTEIN	CARBS	SUGAR	SALT	FIBRE
307kcal	12.3g	4.3g	5.8g	46g	16.9g	1.3g	1.4g

Chocolate Biscuits with Soft Chocolate Centres

This is a great recipe to do with kids, as it's very simple and good fun putting the top circle over the chocolate and squashing the edges gently together to stop the chocolate escaping when it cooks. This is quite a dry mixture, but don't worry, they are meant to look a bit cracked and rustic, so you can't really go wrong! If you eat these warm the chocolate is quite runny, and if you eat them cold they are nice and gooey. You'll need two cutters, one about 4cm and the other about 5cm.

MAKES 30

140g unsalted butter • 140g caster sugar • 2 large egg yolks •
255g self-raising flour • 30g quality cocoa powder • 30 squares
of quality chocolate (milk, white or dark)

Grease a large baking sheet. Cream the butter and sugar together until pale. Beat in the egg yolks, then add the flour and cocoa powder to make a dough. Turn out and knead, then pop it into the fridge to firm up. Preheat the oven to 190°C/375°F/gas 5.

On a lightly floured surface, roll about a third of the dough out thinly, then cut out 30 circles with the smaller cutter (you can do fewer if you want the biscuits bigger). Spread them out on the baking sheet and put a square of the chocolate in the middle of each one – make sure you use all of the chocolate however many you do. Then roll the rest of the dough out (I always add the leftovers from the first lot of cutting to it and knead it a bit). Cut out the same number of circles with the larger cutter and pop them on top of the chocolate, pressing gently all the way round to seal the edge and keep all the chocolate inside.

Bake in the oven for 10 minutes, or until cooked through with a gooey centre. Delicious eaten hot or cold.

CALORIES	FAT	SAT FAT	PROTEIN	CARBS	SUGAR	SALT	FIBRE
24kcal	8.2g	4.8g	1.8g	13.5g	6.9g	0.1g	1.2g

Sticky Toffee Cupcakes with Chocolate Topping

Whatever happened to cupcakes? I used to love them as a kid and, while mucking about with a sticky toffee pudding recipe, I tried to reinvent the good old cupcake – always puts a smile on my face.

MAKES 12

30g sultanas • 30g dried apricots • 30g dates • 1 teaspoon baking powder • 140g self-raising flour • 30g muscovado sugar • 1 tablespoon golden syrup • 1 large egg • 30g unsalted butter

CHOCOLATE TOPPING

40g unsalted butter • 40g caster sugar • 40g quality dark chocolate (70%) • 70ml double cream

Preheat the oven to 200°C/400°F/gas 6. Blitz the sultanas, apricots, dates and baking powder in a food processor with a little of the flour (just enough to stop the fruit sticking to the blades), or chop it very finely by hand. Put this mixture into a bowl with the muscovado sugar, the golden syrup and the egg. Melt the butter, then pour in and stir together. Add 140ml of hot water and the remaining flour and mix well with a whisk. Divide the mixture between 12 cupcake papers (I like to double up the papers to give the mixture a bit more hold) and place on a baking tray. Bake for 15 minutes, or until golden and cooked through.

Meanwhile, melt all the chocolate topping ingredients in a pan and bubble for a while until darkened in colour slightly. Remove from the heat and let the sauce cool until it thickens, then put a blob on top of each cupcake.

CALORIES	FAT	SAT FAT	PROTEIN	CARBS	SUGAR	SALT	FIBRE
127kcal	0.5g	0.1g	4.4g	28g	1.6g	0.4g	1.1g

Frozen Yoghurt

This is almost like ice cream, can be any flavour you like, and is really tasty and refreshing, but more importantly it's so, so quick to make as you don't have to do any whipping or freezing. Just a bit of help from your trusty food processor.

SERVES 4–6

300g frozen fruit, such as strawberries, raspberries, blueberries • 1 x 500g tub of natural yoghurt • optional: runny honey • optional: cornets or wafers

The only important thing to remember here is that your fruit should be in the freezer and frozen and your yoghurt in the fridge and cold before you start. Remove the fruit and place it in your food processor. Blitz for 30 seconds, then add the yoghurt and blend for 1 minute, or until smooth. At this point, taste for sweetness – fruit is normally frozen when it's ripe and at its best, so it should be pretty perfect. If not, add a little honey to taste. It should be scoopable, so eat it straight away or put it into a covered bowl and place in the freezer, where it will keep for a couple of weeks. How good is that?

CALORIES	FAT	SAT FAT	PROTEIN	CARBS	SUGAR	SALT	FIBRE
124kcal	5.3g	3.4g	6.4g	12.8g	12.8g	0.2g	2g

MORE SIMPLE SALADS You'd think there wouldn't be any more salads, or at least any half-decent classy salads left to talk about – but no, we are back with a vengeance. My addiction to the crisp leaf has given me some fantastic ideas which I know you will love. Salads are always great for snacks, lunch or dinner. I've even been known to come back from band practice at two in the morning and do a nice crispy bacon, rocket and Parmesan salad with a bit of balsamic dressing. Not quite a Ruby Murray, but still scrumptious nonetheless. I have also included six fantastic dressings which I know people love – good dressings make good salads even out of a dodgy bit of iceberg lettuce which pretty much tastes of nothing.

I've got a mate called Andy Slade, the local gasman back in Essex, who swears, as a bachelor just moved into his new house, that 'I eat helffy now, Ollie.' I say, 'What do you mean, Andy?' as I look round his kitchen, noticing the plugs and manuals are still in their plastic wrappers inside the oven and washing machine. He replies, 'Well, I always order extra salad in my doner kebab.' What can I say? He needs help … or the love, sympathy and bravery of a good woman!

Andy the gasman

Ollie

Marinated Mozzarella in Crème Fraîche with Lemon & Marjoram

I always love making this salad because it transforms a piece of lovely mozzarella cheese into something really special. In fact, it's classy enough to be a nice starter with a little chopped fresh tomato on some grilled bruschetta.

Simply slice up 4 balls of buffalo mozzarella around 1cm thick, place on a large plate or dish and spread over a small tub or 6 heaped tablespoons of crème fraîche. Season with sea salt and black pepper, to taste. Wash and peel 1 lemon with a speed-peeler and finely chop half the rind. Sprinkle this over the mozzarella and créme fraîche and squeeze over half the juice. Put the leftover lemon to one side in case the flavour needs tweaking later. Sprinkle over a good handful of fresh marjoram leaves. Taste once more for a good balance of flavour.

Halve, deseed and finely slice a couple of fresh red chillies. Sprinkle over the mozzarella, drizzle over 4 tablespoons of extra virgin olive oil, and serve in the middle of the table or as part of another dish. Leftovers will keep for a couple of days in the fridge and are just as scrumptious baked on top of a piece of cod.

CALORIES	FAT	SAT FAT	PROTEIN	CARBS	SUGAR	SALT	FIBRE
300kcal	27.7g	15.5g	12.2g	0.7g	0.7g	0.8g	0.2g

The Easiest Sexiest Salad in the World

SERVES 4

I love this salad. Apart from being a great combination, it always seems unbelievably effortless, which is the kind of recipe I like. The constant success of this is due to the common-sense marriage of salty Parma ham, milky buffalo mozzarella and sweet figs, which obviously need to be of a good quality. The best figs to use are Italian and the best time to buy them is June to August when they are in season. Greek figs are a good second-best and are in season from September to November. The best figs always seem to be those that are about to split their skins. Use green or black figs – it doesn't really matter.

One thing I do is to criss-cross the figs but not quite to the bottom – 1 fig per person is always a good start. Then, using your thumbs and forefingers, squeeze the base of the fig to expose the inside. At this point you'll think, 'Oooh, that looks nice, I think I'm quite clever . . .' or at least I do. More importantly, it allows your dressing to get right into the middle of the fig. All these little things really help to make a salad special. Simply place the figs in a dish, weave around 1 slice of Parma ham or prosciutto per fig, throw in some slices of buffalo mozzarella, rip over some green or purple basil and drizzle everything with Honey & Lemon Juice Dressing (see page 115). As far as salads go, it's pretty damn sexy.

PS Have some spare bread on the table to mop up the juices – always a treat.

CALORIES	FAT	SAT FAT	PROTEIN	CARBS	SUGAR	SALT	FIBRE
242kcal	21.1g	4.3g	5.5g	8g	8g	1g	0.6g

Courgette Salad with Mint, Garlic, Red Chilli, Lemon & Extra Virgin Olive Oil

SERVES 4

This is quite an unusual salad and terribly simple to make. It's great because it's a nice little side dish that will go with things like mozzarella, goat's cheese, cured meats, grilled or barbecued white fish like cod or haddock, even things like chicken or pork. Use courgettes when at their best (nice and firm and not too big).

Slice 4 courgettes lengthways as thin as you can (use a mandolin if you have one – use the guard!). Grill on a red-hot griddle pan, or on the barbecue, until lightly charred on each side. Scatter the slices over a large plate, making sure you don't sit them on top of each other otherwise they'll steam and go a bit limp, and there's nothing worse than limp courgettes, I can tell you. While they're still warmish, sprinkle them with a little sea salt and black pepper.

Deseed 1 fresh red chilli and chop finely. Finely chop ½ a clove of garlic and sprinkle the chilli and garlic evenly from a height over the courgettes. (Add to your own taste, but just remember that when the chilli and garlic mix with the olive oil and lemon juice the heat and flavours are slightly lessened.)

CALORIES	FAT	SAT FAT	PROTEIN	CARBS	SUGAR	SALT	FIBRE
53kcal	2.4g	0.4g	3.8g	4.1g	3.6g	0.3g	1.8g

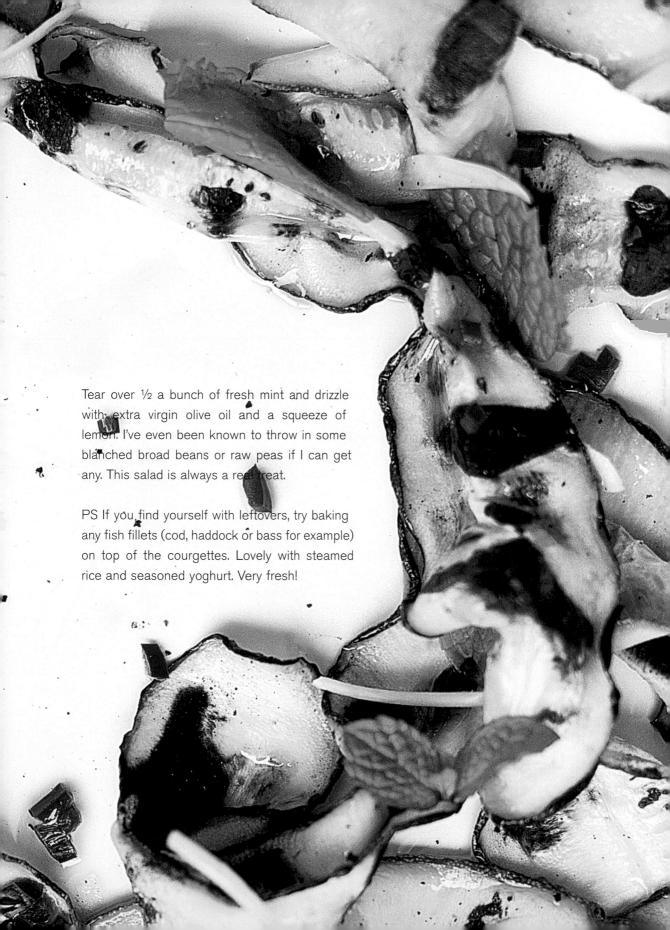

Tear over ½ a bunch of fresh mint and drizzle with extra virgin olive oil and a squeeze of lemon. I've even been known to throw in some blanched broad beans or raw peas if I can get any. This salad is always a real treat.

PS If you find yourself with leftovers, try baking any fish fillets (cod, haddock or bass for example) on top of the courgettes. Lovely with steamed rice and seasoned yoghurt. Very fresh!

Japanese Cucumber Salad with Ginger, Coriander, Mint & Rice Wine Vinegar Dressing

In our supermarkets we have been blessed with a new type of cucumber which is about a third of the size of normal cucumbers. I really like them because they are a touch firmer and ideal for this oriental salad. Wash 3 cucumbers and finely slice along their length with a mandolin (use the guard!) or a speed-peeler. Basically you want to get very fine strips of cucumber. Place the strips on a plate and spread them out. Sprinkle with some ripped-up fresh mint and coriander and drizzle generously with Ginger & Rice Wine Vinegar Dressing (see page 115).

CALORIES	FAT	SAT FAT	PROTEIN	CARBS	SUGAR	SALT	FIBRE
92kcal	8.4g	1.1g	1.5g	2.7g	2.1g	0.2g	1g

Scrummy Warm Rocket Salad

SERVES 4

Warm salads can be blooming amazing or a complete disaster. First, you have got to get your hungry guests around the table before you plate up, so as soon as their bums are on the chairs, you are tossing the warm ingredients in with the rocket leaves. Boom, boom, boom on a plate and it's in front of them.

Peel, halve and quarter 2 medium red onions, then quarter again, to give you 8 pieces from each onion. Heat a frying pan and fry 8 rashers of pancetta or smoked streaky bacon until crisp. Remove to kitchen paper. Drizzle a couple of lugs of olive oil into the pan, and add 4 sprigs of fresh thyme, the onions and a good handful of pine nuts with a pinch of sea salt. Toss around and fry on a medium heat for 5 minutes, or until sweet and caramelized (not black!). Put the pancetta or bacon back into the pan, toss around, then throw everything into a salad bowl with 4 big handfuls of rocket or any nice salad leaves. Drizzle generously with balsamic vinegar – this will make a natural dressing as it mixes with the oil. Serve with some shaved Parmesan – use a speed-peeler to do this. Munch away.

CALORIES	FAT	SAT FAT	PROTEIN	CARBS	SUGAR	SALT	FIBRE
178kcal	14.4g	3.1g	5.6g	6.4g	4.3g	0.8g	1.7g

Japanese Mooli Salad
with Mustard Cress, Crème Fraîche
& Grilled Lemon Dressing

SERVES 4–6

This salad uses fantastic Japanese moolis, which are kind of like oriental radishes. They are crunchy and slightly mustardy in taste and now widely available.

Peel one of these boys and thinly slice it lengthways with a speed-peeler or a mandolin (use the guard!). Once that's done, take 4 or 5 of the slices at a time, line them up together on a chopping board and run your knife down the length of them, cutting them into strips rather like tagliatelle – don't be fussy about getting them exactly the same size. Cutting them into thin strips will help the dressing stick to the mooli, making it taste lovely jubbly.

Mix the mooli strips in a bowl with 3 punnets of mustard cress, tops trimmed, earthy parts binned. Dress with Crème Fraîche & Grilled Lemon Dressing (see page 114) and season well to taste with sea salt and black pepper. Just to get you thinking, in Japan they slice up fine slivers of mango, top-quality raw red mullet and scallops into this salad, which I love – the dressing slightly cures the fish, giving it a nice chewy richness which is great. Give it a bash.

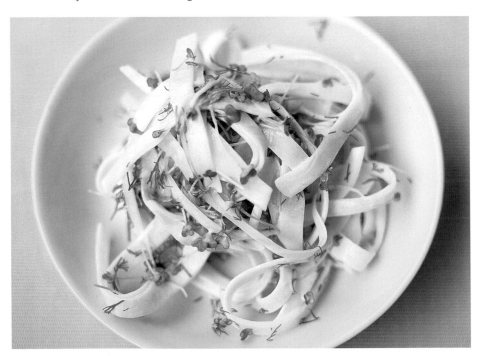

CALORIES	FAT	SAT FAT	PROTEIN	CARBS	SUGAR	SALT	FIBRE
90kcal	7.7g	3g	1.5g	4g	3.9g	0.6g	0.1g

Avocado, Spring Onion, Coriander & Chilli Salad with Toasted Almonds

SERVES 6

Nothing very worldly to say about this salad except it's very tasty. I had a flash of inspiration when looking at my slightly bare fridge and came up with this. It's rather nice with some cold roast chicken, especially in a bit of pitta bread.

Throw a couple of good handfuls of whole blanched almonds into a non-stick pan or tray with the smallest amount of olive oil and toast until lightly golden in the oven, under the grill or over the gas. Whichever way you choose, keep your eyes peeled so they don't burn. Season with sea salt, black pepper and a little dried red chilli and put to one side. You will want 3 avocados, halved, peeled and with the stone removed. Tear the avocado into chunky bits, place in a bowl, sprinkle over 4 or 5 finely sliced spring onions and as much finely sliced fresh green chilli as you like, and rip over ½ a bunch of coriander. Sprinkle over the almonds, drizzle with plenty of Thick Mustard Dressing (see page 114) and season with salt and pepper.

CALORIES	FAT	SAT FAT	PROTEIN	CARBS	SUGAR	SALT	FIBRE
297kcal	30g	5.3g	4.1g	2.9g	1.2g	0.6g	0.7g

A Tuscan Raw Artichoke, Rocket & Parmesan Salad

SERVES 4

When globe artichokes come into season it's always a real treat in Tuscany to be given a bowl of this salad. To prepare the salad, you need one globe artichoke per person. See pages 218–19 for preparation instructions and pictures. Rub the trimmed artichokes with a little lemon to stop them discolouring. Simply slice very finely, then give them a good squeeze of lemon, some extra virgin olive oil, sea salt and black pepper, to taste, and a big handful of rocket. Toss everything together in a bowl and shave over lots of Parmesan cheese, using a speed-peeler or a knife. I love eating this salad on its own before dinner.

CALORIES	FAT	SAT FAT	PROTEIN	CARBS	SUGAR	SALT	FIBRE
62kcal	4g	1.8g	0.2g	2.3g	1.2g	0.4g	0.2g

Globe Artichoke, Pink Grapefruit, Frisée & Pecorino Salad

SERVES 4

For this recipe you could buy good preserved artichokes to save time. If using fresh, whack 8 nice globe artichokes into a large pot of salted water, bring to the boil and cook for around 15 minutes, or until a small knife slides easily into the base (the time will depend on their size). Drain in a colander under running water for a couple of minutes and allow to cool while you segment 2 grapefruits, saving any juice. Place the segments and juice in a bowl with a handful of golden, toasted almonds. Peel off the outer green leaves of the artichokes until you reach the soft and tender yellow ones. With a sharp knife trim off the top and bottom of the artichoke, leaving you with the tender heart. Slice in half and then remove the choke from the middle using a teaspoon. Add the artichokes to the grapefruit and almonds. Drizzle with Honey & Lemon Juice Dressing (see page 115). Add 3 large handfuls of frisée, then toss together. Serve with some shaved pecorino – use a speed-peeler to do this.

CALORIES	FAT	SAT FAT	PROTEIN	CARBS	SUGAR	SALT	FIBRE
199kcal	14.3g	3.1g	8.7g	11.9g	9.4g	0.6g	0.8g

Warm Bread Salad of Crispy Pancetta, Parmesan & Poached Egg

SERVES 4

1 ciabatta loaf • olive oil • 1 clove of garlic, peeled and sliced •
8 slices of pancetta or dry-cured smoked streaky bacon •
1 lemon • extra virgin olive oil • 3 large handfuls of rocket •
1 oak leaf lettuce • 4 large eggs (must be very fresh) •
100g Parmesan cheese, in one piece

Preheat the oven to 200°C/400°F/gas 6. Remove the crusts from the ciabatta, then tear the bread into finger-sized pieces. Place on a baking tray, drizzle with a little olive oil and toss with the garlic and some sea salt and black pepper. Bake for 10 minutes, or until crisp, then lay the pancetta over the bread and bake for 5 more minutes, or until that's crispy too. Mix the lemon juice with 8 tablespoons of extra virgin olive oil and season. Put a big pan of unsalted water on to boil.

In a large bowl, toss the salad leaves, pancetta, bread and dressing together, then divide between 4 plates. When the pan of water is simmering, crack in the 4 eggs. They must be really fresh for successful poached eggs. Cook for 4 minutes for a soft egg, or to your liking. Place an egg on each salad and shave over your Parmesan, using a speed-peeler. Sweeeet!!!

CALORIES	FAT	SAT FAT	PROTEIN	CARBS	SUGAR	SALT	FIBRE
396kcal	19.9g	8.2g	26.4g	29.7g	2.6g	1.9g	2.8g

The Best Pasta Salad

SERVES 4

300g dried small shell-shaped pasta • 3 cloves of garlic •
1 handful of black olives, (stone in) • 250g yellow cherry
tomatoes • ½ a cucumber • 250g red cherry tomatoes •
2 tablespoons fresh chives, finely chopped • 1 bunch of fresh
basil, leaves picked and finely chopped • 4 tablespoons white
wine vinegar, or to taste • extra virgin olive oil

Bring a large pan of salted water to the boil. Throw in the pasta and unpeeled cloves of garlic, boil until al dente, then drain and run under cold water to cool. Put the garlic to one side to use for the dressing. Put the pasta into a bowl. Squash the olives and remove the stones. Chop the tomatoes, olives and cucumber into pieces about half the size of the pasta and add to the bowl with the chives and basil. Squash the garlic cloves out of their skins and mush in a pestle and mortar. Add the vinegar, 6 tablespoons of oil and season with sea salt and black pepper. Drizzle this over the salad, adding a little more seasoning to taste.

CALORIES	FAT	SAT FAT	PROTEIN	CARBS	SUGAR	SALT	FIBRE
471kcal	21.6g	4.4g	11.1g	61.7g	7.2g	1.1g	4.4g

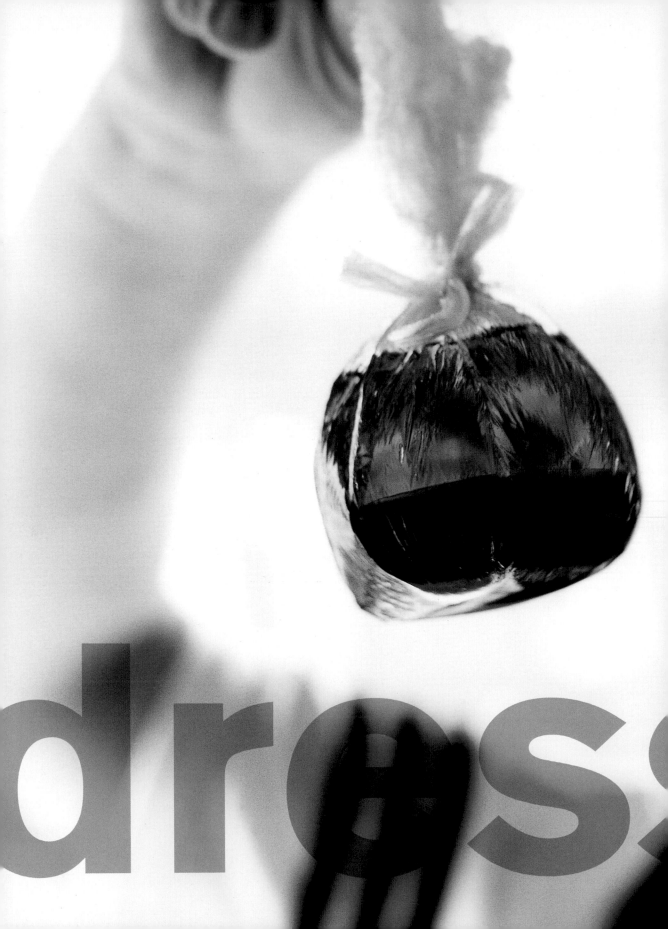

dress

ings

Herb Vinegar & Roasted Garlic Dressing

3 cloves of garlic, unpeeled, roasted or boiled until soft •
6 tablespoons extra virgin olive oil • 1 heaped teaspoon Dijon
mustard • 3 tablespoons good herb vinegar, red or white

Squeeze the garlic out of its skin, mush up and mix in a bowl with the rest of the
ingredients, then season to taste with sea salt and black pepper.

CALORIES	FAT	SAT FAT	PROTEIN	CARBS	SUGAR	SALT	FIBRE
85kcal	7.9g	1.1g	1.1g	2.2g	0.2g	0.2g	0g

Crème Fraîche & Grilled Lemon Dressing

1 large lemon, halved • 3 tablespoons extra virgin olive oil •
3 tablespoons crème fraîche or mayonnaise • 2 heaped
teaspoons Dijon mustard • low-salt soy sauce

Grill the lemon halves on a griddle pan for 5 minutes, or until soft and
charred, then squeeze the juice into a bowl. Mix with the rest of the ingredients,
then season to taste with soy sauce and black pepper.

CALORIES	FAT	SAT FAT	PROTEIN	CARBS	SUGAR	SALT	FIBRE
71kcal	7.6g	3g	0.4g	0.4g	0.3g	0.2g	0g

Thick Mustard Dressing

6 tablespoons extra virgin olive oil • 2 heaped tablespoons
Dijon mustard • 1 heaped tablespoon wholegrain mustard •
2 tablespoons white wine vinegar

Mix all the ingredients together in a bowl, then season to taste with
sea salt and black pepper.

CALORIES	FAT	SAT FAT	PROTEIN	CARBS	SUGAR	SALT	FIBRE
70kcal	7.6g	1.1g	0.3g	0.1g	0.1g	0.4g	0g

Honey & Lemon Juice Dressing

6 tablespoons extra virgin olive oil • 3 tablespoons
lemon juice • 1 tablespoon runny honey

Mix all the ingredients together in a bowl, then season to taste with
sea salt and black pepper.

CALORIES	FAT	SAT FAT	PROTEIN	CARBS	SUGAR	SALT	FIBRE
71kcal	7.1g	1g	0g	1.7g	1.7g	0.2g	0g

Ginger & Rice Wine Vinegar Dressing

6 tablespoons extra virgin olive oil • 3 tablespoons rice wine
vinegar • 1 teaspoon sugar • 5cm piece of ginger, peeled and
finely grated • 1 stick of lemongrass, outer leaves removed,
inner ones finely chopped • low-salt soy sauce

Mix all the ingredients together in a bowl, then season to taste with
soy sauce and black pepper.

CALORIES	FAT	SAT FAT	PROTEIN	CARBS	SUGAR	SALT	FIBRE
75kcal	7.8g	1.1g	0.1g	1g	0.6g	0.4g	0.1g

Bashed-up Pine Nut, Basil & Balsamic Dressing

½ a clove of garlic, peeled and bashed to a pulp • 1 bunch of
fresh basil, bashed to a pulp • 1 small handful of toasted pine
nuts, bashed to bits • 6 tablespoons extra virgin olive oil •
3 tablespoons balsamic vinegar

Mix all the ingredients together in a bowl, then season to taste with
sea salt and black pepper.

CALORIES	FAT	SAT FAT	PROTEIN	CARBS	SUGAR	SALT	FIBRE
143kcal	14.4g	2g	0.5g	2.7g	2.5g	0.3g	0.1g

Gennaro

Curly

pa

Mauro

PASTA No matter what I do, where I go or who I meet, pasta always comes through with flying colours as one of my favourite regular meals. So I've put together some superb little pasta dishes which will see you through from comfort food to dinner parties. This time I've used mostly dried pasta, as it's so convenient and cheap. Don't be fooled into thinking that fresh pasta is the best — it's just different. Fresh pasta lends itself better to creamy, buttery sauces, while dried pasta is better with tomato and olive oil based sauces. If, however, you do fancy making fresh pasta, then take a look at my two earlier books.

Spaghetti with Sweet Cherry Tomatoes, Marjoram & Extra Virgin Olive Oil

When tomatoes are good, this is super nice. It's a warm dish as opposed to hot, but is even great when cold as a salad for picnics.

SERVES 6

450g dried spaghetti, spaghettini or linguine • 400g ripe cherry tomatoes, ideally red and yellow • 1 bunch of fresh marjoram or basil, leaves picked • 6 tablespoons extra virgin olive oil • 1 clove of garlic, peeled and finely sliced • 1 tablespoon white or red wine vinegar

Cook the pasta in a large pan of boiling salted water according to the packet instructions. While it's cooking, halve the tomatoes, put them into a large bowl, and add the herbs, oil, garlic and vinegar. Season to taste with sea salt and black pepper, and scrunch with your hands to slightly mush the tomatoes — this can sit until the pasta's ready. Drain the pasta, and while still steaming hot mix well with the tomatoes, check the seasoning and serve. Easy peasy.

CALORIES	FAT	SAT FAT	PROTEIN	CARBS	SUGAR	SALT	FIBRE
381kcal	13.4g	1.9g	9.4g	59.4g	4g	0.2g	0.9g

Spaghetti with Salami, Fennel & Tomatoes

SERVES 6

olive oil • 140g quality spicy Italian salami, sliced •
2 cloves of garlic, peeled and finely sliced •
1 teaspoon fennel seeds • 1 bulb of fennel, halved and
finely sliced, herby tops reserved and chopped •
2 x 400g tins of quality plum tomatoes • optional: 1 dried
red chilli, crumbled • 450g dried spaghetti or linguine •
2 handfuls of stale breadcrumbs • optional: 1 sprig of
fresh rosemary

Pour 2 good lugs of oil into a pan, and add the salami and sliced garlic. Lightly crack the fennel seeds either in a pestle and mortar or with a knife and add to the pan. Cook for 1 minute on a low heat – the fat should cook out of the salami and it should begin to crisp up. Add the sliced fennel and stir well, then put the lid on and up the heat to medium. Cook for 5 minutes, then add the tomatoes, breaking them up with a wooden spoon, and even a little dried chilli, if you like. Cook slowly for 25 minutes, or until the mixture has thickened. Season to taste with sea salt and black pepper.

Cook the pasta in a large pan of boiling salted water according to the packet instructions. While it's cooking, I like to make pangrattato (crunchy breadcrumbs), to give this dish a great texture and crunch. Just get a couple of good handfuls of coarse breadcrumbs – I do this by removing the crusts from some stale bread and whizzing them up until kind of coarse in a food processor. Fry with 4 or 5 tablespoons of oil until crisp. Sometimes I throw in some rosemary sprigs for extra flavour. Drain the pasta, and immediately toss with the lovely tomato sauce. This is quite rich but very very tasty.

Serve in a large bowl and sprinkle with the herby fennel tops and some crispy pangrattato. Eat immediately, with a good glass of red wine.

PS I've eaten a couple of pasta dishes similar to this in Tuscany. Sometimes really good sausages or sliced, cured salamis are used. It's quite a hearty pasta, but the fennel does cut through and makes it a little fresher and more delicate.

CALORIES	FAT	SAT FAT	PROTEIN	CARBS	SUGAR	SALT	FIBRE
433kcal	13.7g	4g	15.5g	65.6g	5.8g	1.2g	1g

Kinda Spaghetti Bolognese

As far as I know, no decent Italian cook has any real recollection of what we know as Spaghetti Bolognese. However, every region in Italy makes its own ragù, which very often features leftover stewed meats and game. For a great bolognese it's worth whizzing up some chopped chuck steak to make your own minced meat. Here's my version – I hope you like it.

SERVES 6

10 slices of pancetta or smoked streaky bacon, finely sliced • ½ a bunch of fresh rosemary, leaves picked and roughly chopped • olive oil • 1 large onion, peeled and finely chopped • 3 cloves of garlic, peeled and finely chopped • 450g chuck steak, minced, or quality minced beef • 1 wineglass of red wine • 1 level teaspoon dried oregano • 1 x 400g tin of quality plum tomatoes • 1 x 200g tube of tomato purée or 1 small jar of sun-dried tomatoes, finely chopped • 450g dried spaghetti • 1 bunch of fresh basil, leaves picked • 2 handfuls of freshly grated Parmesan or mature Cheddar cheese

Preheat the oven to 180°C/350°F/gas 4. In a large hot ovenproof pan, fry the pancetta and rosemary in a little oil until lightly golden. Add the onion and garlic and fry for a further 3 minutes, or until softened, before adding the minced beef. Stir and continue frying for 2 or 3 minutes before adding the wine. Reduce slightly, then add the oregano, all the tomatoes, breaking them up with a wooden spoon, and the tomato purée. Season with sea salt and black pepper, bring to the boil, then cover with greaseproof paper or a lid, and place in the oven for 1 hour 30 minutes, or until thickened and reduced. Towards the end of the cooking time, cook the pasta in a large pan of boiling salted water according to the packet instructions, then drain.

Just before serving, tear the basil into the sauce. Serve with the spaghetti and some grated cheese. Delicious served with a green salad.

CALORIES	FAT	SAT FAT	PROTEIN	CARBS	SUGAR	SALT	FIBRE
566kcal	19.3g	8.1g	30g	67.2g	10.8g	0.8g	3.3g

Honeymoon Spaghetti

I first tried this at Hotel St Pietro in Positano, Italy, where Jools and I stayed for a week of our honeymoon. The steam will cause the parcel to puff up in the oven, which looks good at the table if you serve it straight away. My dad hasn't stopped cooking it – maybe he's got a second wind – the little tiger!

SERVES 6

1 x 1.5kg crab or lobster • 2 cloves of garlic, peeled and chopped • 1 fresh red chilli, deseeded and finely sliced • 30g unsalted butter • olive oil • 450g mussels, scrubbed, debearded • 100g squid, sliced • 200g raw shell-off tiger or small prawns • 450g dried spaghetti, cooked al dente • 1 bunch of fresh flat-leaf parsley and marjoram, picked and roughly chopped • 1 large egg, beaten

SAUCE

olive oil • 3 cloves of garlic, peeled and roughly chopped • 1 fresh red chilli, finely chopped • 2 x 400g tins of quality plum tomatoes

Preheat the oven to 180°C/350°F/gas 4. Plunge the crab or lobster into boiling water and boil for 15 minutes, then remove. Once cooled, remove all the meat from the shell, flaking it up into small pieces, and removing any splinters of shell.

To make the sauce, fry the empty shell and legs in 1 tablespoon of oil with the garlic and chilli. Pound up the shells using a rolling pin. Add the tomatoes, breaking them up with a wooden spoon, and a large glass of water and simmer for 1 hour. Pass through a sieve and season to taste with sea salt and black pepper.

In a large pan, gently fry the garlic and chilli from the main list in the butter and 1 tablespoon of oil. Turn the heat up and add the mussels, squid and prawns. Cook for 2 minutes. Remove from the heat, discarding any unopened mussels. Add the tomato sauce, cooked pasta, crab or lobster meat and herbs, then mix together.

Fold a 60cm x 120cm piece of greaseproof in half to get a crease and open it out again. Place the seafood mixture in the centre of one half and brush all the edges with beaten egg. Bring the two sides together and seal well. Carefully slide the parcel on to a baking tray and cook for 10 minutes, or until puffed up.

CALORIES	FAT	SAT FAT	PROTEIN	CARBS	SUGAR	SALT	FIBRE
476kcal	10.9g	3.7g	34.8g	64g	7g	1.2g	1.1g

Penne Carbonara

This is the way it should be done, guys. Simple, quick and cheap – happy days.

SERVES 6

450g dried penne • 10 slices of pancetta or dry-cured smoked streaky bacon • olive oil • 5 large egg yolks • 100ml double cream • 125g Parmesan cheese, freshly grated

Cook the pasta in boiling salted water according to the packet instructions. While it's cooking, slowly fry the pancetta in a little oil until crispy. Break it up a bit, then put to one side. Whip up the egg yolks, cream and half the Parmesan. Drain the pasta and immediately toss with the warm, crispy pancetta and the egg mixture. A lot of carbonaras are over-cooked and resemble a scrambled egg sauce – if you add the pasta immediately the residual heat is enough to cook the eggs and for the sauce to stay smooth and silky. Season well with sea salt and plenty of black pepper, and add extra Parmesan, to taste. Serve straight away, with a big bowl of salad and a nice bottle of red wine, if you like.

CALORIES	FAT	SAT FAT	PROTEIN	CARBS	SUGAR	SALT	FIBRE
514kcal	24.2g	12g	20.5g	57.2g	2g	0.8g	0g

Open Lasagne of Sweet Tomatoes, Squid, Mussels, Farro & Olives

This dish is a real joy, inspired by a great American chef called Mario Bartelli who made me a simple squid stew on one of my trips to America. He called it 'two-minute squid' and it has stayed in my memory ever since. I've changed it slightly so that it is now a pukka pasta dish, but it can be thinned slightly with a little stock to make a great soup, or you can use it as a sauce over some grilled fish. Tossed with lasagne, like this, or with some tagliatelle, it's brilliant. Farro is a grain, similar to couscous or bulgur wheat, which has a great nutty flavour.

SERVES 6

1 red onion, peeled and finely chopped • 2 cloves of garlic, peeled and finely sliced • olive oil • 2 handfuls of black olives (stone in) • 50g farro • 2 x 400g tins of quality plum tomatoes • 400g mussels, scrubbed, debearded • 400g clams • 300g squid, gutted, cleaned, sliced • 12 fresh lasagne sheets • 1 bunch of fresh flat-leaf parsley, leaves picked and chopped • extra virgin olive oil

In a large pot, slowly fry the onion and garlic in a little olive oil for 1 minute, while you squash and destone the olives. Add the farro, olives and tomatoes, breaking them up with a wooden spoon, and simmer for 30 minutes. Add the mussels and clams and shake around until they all open up (discard any that remain closed), then add the squid and simmer for 1 minute. Remove the meat from most of the shells, then cook the pasta in boiling salted water according to the packet instructions. Season the sauce carefully with sea salt and black pepper, throw in the parsley, and stir through 5 tablespoons of extra virgin olive oil to give it a good shine. Drain the pasta and immediately toss with the sauce, then serve.

CALORIES	FAT	SAT FAT	PROTEIN	CARBS	SUGAR	SALT	FIBRE
482kcal	14.8g	2.4g	27.4g	63.1g	8.8g	0.8g	5.1g

Parsnip & Pancetta Tagliatelle with Parmesan & Butter

I'd never thought of the parsnip and pancetta combination until about a year ago – slightly unusual, but what a great combo. It's bloody good and I've used them together ever since in soups, risottos, roasts and casseroles.

SERVES 6

8 slices of pancetta or dry-cured smoked streaky bacon • 1 bunch of fresh rosemary, thyme or summer savory, leaves picked • 4 good knobs of unsalted butter • 2 cloves of garlic, peeled and finely sliced • 2 parsnips, peeled, halved and finely sliced lengthways • 450g dried tagliatelle • 3 good handfuls of freshly grated Parmesan cheese

Fry the pancetta and herbs in a large non-stick frying pan on a medium heat with half the butter for 2 minutes, then add the garlic and parsnips. Cook for a further 3 minutes, or until the pancetta is slightly golden and the parsnips have softened nicely. Cook the pasta in boiling salted water according to the packet instructions, then drain, reserving a little of the cooking water. Mix the pasta with the parsnips and pancetta and stir in the remaining butter and the Parmesan, adding a little of the cooking water to loosen and make it creamy and shiny. Season to taste with sea salt and black pepper, then serve up.

CALORIES	FAT	SAT FAT	PROTEIN	CARBS	SUGAR	SALT	FIBRE
393kcal	11.2g	6g	13.9g	63.1g	4.4g	0.6g	0.3g

Broccoli & Anchovy Orecchiette

You must try this one. Penne and rigatoni work well in place of orecchiette – and are widely available everywhere.

SERVES 6

2 large heads of broccoli • 2 large cloves of garlic, peeled and chopped • 8 anchovy fillets, in oil • 2–4 small dried red chillies, crumbled, to your taste • 4 good knobs of butter • 450g dried orecchiette • 2 good handfuls of freshly grated Parmesan cheese

Using a small knife, trim round the broccoli to remove the dark green florets from the main stalks and put them to one side. Peel the stalks, trim off the dry end and throw this away. Finely chop the stalk and put into a large pan with the garlic, anchovies, chillies and half the butter. Cover with a lid and cook slowly for 8 to 10 minutes while you cook the pasta in boiling salted water according to the packet instructions. Something I like to do which is slightly different (but better, I'd like to think) is to cook the broccoli florets with the pasta for the last 4 minutes – this makes them soft enough to eat but leaves them with great colour and texture.

Drain the pasta and broccoli, saving a little of the cooking water, then toss into the other pan. Remove the pan from the heat. Season to taste with sea salt, black pepper, the rest of the butter and a large handful of Parmesan. Mix well, adding a little of the cooking water, to loosen, if needed, and make it shine. Serve immediately, sprinkled with the rest of the Parmesan.

CALORIES	FAT	SAT FAT	PROTEIN	CARBS	SUGAR	SALT	FIBRE
367kcal	9.5g	5.1g	14.8g	59.4g	3g	1.3g	2.4g

Show time: Jamie Oliver, 25, has an energy that has made him a TV star and a hot cookbook author.

By Alastair Grant for USA TODAY

Brit's a rock star in chef's clothing

TV's 'Naked' sensation serves up books – and lif...

SOMETHING FISHY GOING ON Fish is a fantastic thing. When you look at the way the Spanish, Italians and Japanese live and at their statistics of life expectancy, their consumption of fish seems to play a large part. I don't think any doctor has ever ruled out the fact that fish is really, really good for your diet. So if you are a grumpy bugger, or you're married to one, who will only eat fish in batter, hopefully this chapter will be enough to twist your arm. Not only does fresh fish need minimal cooking, but it's damn tasty too. Think of your taste buds, think of your heart and do yourself a favour – eat fresh fish at least twice a week. When buying fish you should trust your own instincts and go for ones that look, feel and smell really good. It's also quite wise to become chummy with your fishmonger – find out when the freshest fish comes in, then make sure he reserves it for you.

Whole Roasted Salmon Wrapped in Herbs & Newspaper

Absolutely great for parties, this recipe is a fantastic way to cook pretty much any whole fish, particularly salmon and trout. It's best cooked on a camp fire, over a barbecue or in a wood oven, as the paper will begin to burn, giving you a subtle smoked flavour. You will still get great results from cooking in a conventional oven but the newspaper will not blacken as on a camp fire. This recipe varies very little, depending on the number of people that you want to serve – for more than 6, just use a bigger salmon, more herbs, more paper and a slightly longer cooking time.

SERVES 6

1 x 1.5kg whole salmon, skin on, scaled, gutted • olive oil •
4 bunches of mixed fresh herbs, such as flat-leaf parsley, fennel
tops, basil • a copy of *The Times* (or your regular paper!) •
2 lemons, thinly sliced • 6 spring onions, thinly sliced •
2 tablespoons fennel seeds, cracked

Season the salmon inside and out with sea salt and black pepper, then rub with oil and stuff with half the herbs. Open the paper out to the middle page, then place a large sheet of greaseproof paper on top and place the salmon in the centre. Scatter over the lemons, spring onions, fennel seeds and remaining herbs. Tuck some of these underneath and over the salmon. Drizzle with a little extra oil, tuck in the sides of the paper and fold to wrap up tightly, securing it well with lots of string. Wet the paper really well under the tap and either place directly on a shelf at the top of the oven, preheated to 220°C/425°F/gas 7, for 35 minutes, or preferably cook on the barbie or on a rack over a camp fire for about 25 minutes on each side, depending on the intensity of the heat.

Salmon is a good fish for this recipe because it's quite fatty, so whether it's still a bit pink or slightly overdone it's still very acceptable. I like it slightly pink, served with some boiled potatoes, green salad and homemade mayonnaise – fantastic.

CALORIES	FAT	SAT FAT	PROTEIN	CARBS	SUGAR	SALT	FIBRE
334kcal	21.5g	3.9g	35.2g	1.5g	1.3g	0.4g	0g

Essex Oysters Freshly Shucked on Bashed-up Ice – My Favourite Ways

Oysters are funny old things. Now they're considered a decadent aphrodisiac, when only 100 years ago they were the pigeons of the sea and would be chucked into pies as peasant food. Aphrodisiac? I'm not sure, but I do seem to have acquired a taste for them over the last 3 years.

I've eaten oysters all round the world and everyone seems to think that theirs are the best – well, I'll join the patriotic club and say that the best oysters I've ever eaten in my life are West Mersea Essex native oysters, sometimes known as Colchester oysters, along with some West Irish oysters that have a beautiful iron and subtle seawatery taste. The oysters directly from West Mersea are fantastic because they are farmed a couple of miles down the estuary where Maldon sea salt comes from. The nutrients from the marshland are leached out when the rain falls on it and are later drained into the estuary, so it's a fantastically nutritious area. I'll always go for small oysters because, quite frankly, I can't handle the big ones.

But no matter what kind of oysters you have, here's two fantastic ways to knock them back. You can get your fishmonger to open the oysters for you or you can freshly shuck (open) them with a small knife or oyster-shucker, using a tea towel to hold them (see pictures opposite), eat them the day that you buy them and serve them on some ice cubes that you've bashed up in a tea towel.

Find pointed pivot joint

2. Push and wiggle in the shucker

3. Twist and prise open the shell

4. Remove shell and loosen the oyster

Oysters with Shallots & Red Wine Vinegar

Finely chop 1 peeled shallot and mix with 2 heaped teaspoons of sugar, 6 tablespoons of red wine vinegar and a little black pepper. Allow to sit for 10 minutes. Serve in a dish with a load of oysters.

CALORIES	FAT	SAT FAT	PROTEIN	CARBS	SUGAR	SALT	FIBRE
38kcal	0.6g	0.1g	5.2g	2.6g	1.3g	0.6g	0.1g

Oysters with Chilli, Ginger & Rice Wine Vinegar

Finely grate a 2.5cm thumb-sized piece of peeled ginger and mix with
6 tablespoons of rice wine vinegar, 1 finely chopped and deseeded
fresh red chilli and a little finely sliced fresh
coriander. Stir in 1 teaspoon of
sugar until dissolved. Serve
in a dish with a load
of oysters.

CALORIES	FAT	SAT FAT	PROTEIN	CARBS	SUGAR	SALT	FIBRE
36kcal	0.7g	0.1g	5.3g	2.2g	0.7g	0.6g	0.1g

Seared Tuna
with Grated Ginger & Chives

This is pretty much simplicity at its best. I had this in a sushi bar in Tokyo and loved being able to appreciate the deep red fresh tuna. It is just a matter of very quickly searing the fish, then mopping it through a little soy sauce, ginger and chives and whopping it straight in your choppers.

SERVES 4

250g tuna, preferably the tail end or a thin strip of the loin •
low-salt soy sauce • 1 tablespoon groundnut oil •
10cm piece of ginger • 1 bunch of fresh chives, finely sliced

Marinate the tuna in a little soy sauce for 1 hour. Pat dry, rub with oil and sear for around 2 minutes in a very hot non-stick frying pan, turning regularly. Allow to sit for 1 minute while you peel and finely grate the ginger. To serve, place a little blob of ginger and a small pile of chives on one side of each plate, with a pool of soy sauce in the middle. Using a sharp knife, cut the tuna into ½–1cm thick slices, giving each person at least 3 or 4 pieces. In Japan, thicker slices are considered a sign of generosity and real decadence, but I still like them quite thin.

CALORIES	FAT	SAT FAT	PROTEIN	CARBS	SUGAR	SALT	FIBRE
110kcal	3.7g	0.6g	17.4g	1.7g	0.6g	1.2g	0.2g

Sicilian Roasted Brill Steak
with Lemon, Anchovies, Capers & Rosemary

This is a fantastic way to eat meaty white fish like brill, turbot and halibut. It's really special if they're cut through the bone into tranches (steaks) – a nice fillet will do as well. Ask your fishmonger to cut the steaks for you. You can get hold of Sicilian lemons in some supermarkets now.

SERVES 4

½ a bunch of fresh rosemary, leaves picked • olive oil •
4 x 200g brill, turbot or halibut tranches • 2 large lemons,
finely sliced • 1 large handful of baby capers • 8 good anchovy
fillets, in oil • 1 splash of white wine or prosecco

Preheat the oven to 200°C/400°F/gas 6. Bruise the rosemary in a pestle and mortar to bring out the flavour. Add 6 tablespoons of oil and scrunch together. Pat half the flavoured oil around the fish, season well with sea salt and black pepper and put into an earthenware dish or roasting tray. Lay 4 or 5 thin slices of lemon over each steak (I normally slice these on a mandolin – use the guard! – or use a very sharp knife). Sprinkle over the capers, and drape over the anchovies. Drizzle with the remaining flavoured oil and bake for 15 minutes off the bone or 25 minutes on the bone. Now splash in a little wine, then remove from the oven and allow to rest, just like a steak, for 5 minutes. Sometimes I like to squeeze a little extra lemon juice over the fish so it can mix with the white creamy cooking juice and oil, making an amazing natural sauce. Great served with any steamed seasonal greens or a good crisp salad.

CALORIES	FAT	SAT FAT	PROTEIN	CARBS	SUGAR	SALT	FIBRE
378kcal	24.1g	4.1g	37.5g	1.9g	1.5g	1.9g	0.4g

Rosemary Skewered Monkfish with Pancetta & Bread

This is a forever-winning combo that involves the slightly unusual marriage between meat and fish. It works out pretty cost-effective as well, because you're using less fish than you normally would and you're actually making it taste a lot more interesting too. Give it a bash.

SERVES 4

450g monkfish fillets, skin off (or any meaty white fish) •
1½ ciabatta loaves, crusts removed • 4 x 25cm fresh rosemary
twigs • 1 clove of garlic, peeled • olive oil • 12 slices of
pancetta or dry-cured smoked streaky bacon • 1–2 tablespoons
good balsamic vinegar • extra virgin olive oil

Preheat the oven to 220°C/425°F/gas 7. Cut the monkfish into 2.5cm dice and place in a bowl with the ciabatta, ripped up into similar-sized pieces. Keeping the top 5cm of rosemary leaves, run your thumb and forefinger down the length of the twigs, removing all the leaves. Throw these into a pestle and mortar and bash up with the garlic, then stir in 5 or 6 tablespoons of olive oil. Pour this over the monkfish and bread and toss to coat.

Now begin to skewer the kebabs. At an angle, slice the tip off the rosemary stalks, so they are sharp. Put a piece of monkfish on first, then bread, and repeat until you have about 3 pieces of monkfish and about 3 pieces of bread on each kebab and lightly season with sea salt and black pepper. Loosely wrap 3 pieces of pancetta round each kebab, weaving it in and around the fish and the bread. Place the kebabs on a roasting tray, sprinkle with any leftover oil and rosemary, and bake in the oven for 15 to 20 minutes, or until the bread is golden and crisp. Drizzle a little balsamic vinegar over each piece of monkfish, then a little extra virgin olive oil and any juices from the tray. Serve simply with a good salad. Happy days!

CALORIES	FAT	SAT FAT	PROTEIN	CARBS	SUGAR	SALT	FIBRE
444kcal	22g	4.1g	26.7g	36.9g	3.2g	1.1g	2.8g

Prawns with Chilli, Parsley, Ginger & Garlic on Toast

This is a really quick dinner which always hits the spot. Nice to do as a starter, too. Just put some finger-bowls on the table and let your mates dive in. I always put a little extra chilli in and make sure I've got some nice cold wine on the go as well.

SERVES 4

olive oil • 5cm piece of ginger, peeled and finely chopped • 2 cloves of garlic, peeled and finely sliced • 2–3 fresh red chillies, deseeded and finely sliced • 16 large raw peeled tiger prawns, tails left on or off • 1–2 lemons, to taste • 1 bunch of fresh flat-leaf parsley, leaves picked and roughly chopped • 4 long slices of ciabatta, toasted

Drizzle 4 tablespoons of oil into a large, hot frying pan and add the ginger, garlic, chillies and prawns. Fry for about 3 minutes, then turn the heat down and squeeze in the juice of 1 lemon. Add the parsley and a couple of lugs of oil. Toss over and remove from the heat. You should have a nice juicy sauce – have a taste, it may need a little more lemon juice. Season to taste with sea salt and black pepper. Serve over the ciabatta, to mop up the juices.

CALORIES	FAT	SAT FAT	PROTEIN	CARBS	SUGAR	SALT	FIBRE
244kcal	13.6g	2g	15.2g	16.3g	1.3g	0.9g	1.1g

Lovely Traybaked Plaice
with Spinach, Olives & Tomatoes

Another great traybaked recipe, which is perfect for coping with lots of people without a huge deal of effort. You can use any similar flat fish, like lemon sole, instead of plaice, if you prefer.

SERVES 4

olive oil • 2 cloves of garlic, peeled and sliced •
1 wineglass of Chardonnay • 2 x 400g tins of quality plum
tomatoes • 150g black olives, stone in • 1 big bunch of fresh
basil • 2 anchovy fillets, in oil • 4 x 200g plaice fillets, skin off •
4 fresh rosemary twigs or cocktail sticks • 3 large handfuls
of baby spinach

Preheat the oven to 200°C/400°F/gas 6. Use a small roasting tray, so the fish cooks snugly. Put the tray over a medium heat on the hob, add a little oil, and slowly fry the garlic until softened. Before it colours, add the wine and cook for 1 minute, then add the tomatoes, breaking them up with a wooden spoon, and turn down to a simmer while you prepare the plaice.

Squash the olives and remove the stones, then finely chop or purée with the basil and anchovy fillets in a food processor. Add oil to loosen, giving you a spreadable paste. On a board, lay the plaice fillets down on what was their skin side and season with black pepper. Divide the paste into 4 and spread all over the fillets. Roll each fillet up like a Swiss roll from the tail end and secure with a spiked piece of rosemary, or a cocktail stick, to hold it together. Season the tomato sauce with sea salt and black pepper, then place the fish fillets next to each other on top of the sauce. Drizzle with oil and bake in the oven for 15 minutes – the sauce will flavour the plaice and vice versa, which is great.

Remove the fish to 4 warmed plates and place the sauce back on the hob for 1 minute, while you throw in the spinach – it will wilt quickly. Spoon the spinachy sauce next to the fish and get stuck in. Beautiful.

CALORIES	FAT	SAT FAT	PROTEIN	CARBS	SUGAR	SALT	FIBRE
295kcal	7.6g	1.2g	36.8g	12.9g	7.9g	2.1g	3.6g

Magnificent Roasted Monkfish

The whole idea behind this recipe was to be able to make something really quick and ultra-tasty and present it in a way that looked like you'd been working for hours on it. As monkfish comes in different sizes, feel free to do individual 200g fillets or to cook a whole larger fillet and divide it up once cooked. So, here goes.

SERVES 4

1 small jar of sun-dried tomatoes, in oil • 1 big bunch
of fresh basil • olive oil • 16 slices of Parma ham • 4 x 200g
monkfish tail fillets, trimmed • optional: balsamic vinegar
and rocket, to serve

Preheat the oven to 200°C/400°F/gas 6. Place the sun-dried tomatoes and half their flavoursome preserving oil in a food processor with the basil and blitz until smooth. While blending, I add the remaining preserving oil to the paste until it's nice and spreadable. Sometimes even a dash of balsamic vinegar is quite nice to flavour and loosen it up a bit.

You're going to need 4 x A4-sized pieces of greaseproof paper. Rub some oil over each piece and lay about 4 slices of Parma ham snugly next to each other, on each. Divide the paste into 4, spreading each part evenly over the ham. Place the monkfish fillets at one end, season with sea salt and black pepper, and, using the paper, fold and roll up. Remove the paper and carefully move to an oiled baking tray or dish, then roast in the oven for 15 to 20 minutes.

I like to slice the fish up and serve it with some really buttery mashed potato, thinned down with lots of milk. And maybe drizzle a little balsamic vinegar over the fish, and scatter a little rocket over the whole plate.

CALORIES	FAT	SAT FAT	PROTEIN	CARBS	SUGAR	SALT	FIBRE
359kcal	13.1g	3.5g	50.1g	9.9g	4.5g	4.6g	1.8g

Fried & Roasted Skate Wings
with Lemon & Five-spice Salt

There's nothing better than a good piece of fresh skate but this method of cooking always cheers me up. It's still as moreish and lovely as skate always is, but the lemon and five-spice liven it up and make it quite exciting. A good little trick is to use a pair of scissors or a sharp knife and remove the flimsy edges of the wings, as these will only curl up and burn anyway.

SERVES 4

1 lemon • 1 teaspoon Chinese five-spice • 4 x 225g
skate or ray wings, trimmed • 2 handfuls of plain flour, for
dusting • 2 large eggs, beaten • 6 good handfuls of fine
breadcrumbs • olive oil

Preheat the oven to 220°C/425°F/gas 7. Finely grate the lemon zest into a pestle and mortar. Add the five-spice and 1 heaped teaspoon of sea salt, bash up and mix, then sprinkle over both sides of the wings. Get 3 large plates and put the flour on one, the eggs on another and the breadcrumbs on the third. Put a large non-stick pan on a high heat and add 1cm of oil. Working quickly, dip both sides of each wing first into the flour, shaking off any excess, then into the eggs, allowing the excess to drip off. Next press firmly into the breadcrumbs, shaking off the excess.

Fry the skate wings, either 1 or 2 at a time, in hot oil for 2 minutes on each side, or until lightly golden. Place on a large roasting tray while you fry the remaining fish, changing the oil, if necessary. When all 4 skate wings are done, place the roasting tray in the middle of the oven for 15 minutes, by which time the fish should be golden and crisp and the meat should just pull away from the bone.

I like to serve this with a light herb salad and a dollop of flavoured mayonnaise. Simply mix 4 tablespoons of mayonnaise, or crème fraîche, with 2 handfuls of chopped spring onions, chopped fresh coriander and lime juice, to taste.

CALORIES	FAT	SAT FAT	PROTEIN	CARBS	SUGAR	SALT	FIBRE
652kcal	34.5g	5.3g	43.9g	41.3g	3.6g	2.6g	2.8g

Pan-seared Scallops
with Asparagus & Baby Leeks

I've come across a couple of fantastic revelations that I want to tell you about. First, by scoring the scallops on one side in a criss-cross fashion they open out when seared like a beautiful flower and when dressed they take in all the flavour. Second, the subtle use of five-spice with any seafood is a real pleasure.

SERVES 4

16 asparagus spears, trimmed • 12 baby leeks, washed and trimmed • olive oil • 1 bunch of fresh marjoram or summer savory, leaves picked • 1 lemon • 12 large scallops, trimmed • 2 pinches of Chinese five-spice • unsalted butter

Blanch the asparagus and leeks in boiling salted water for a couple of minutes, or until just tender, then drain. Get a large, non-stick frying pan hot, then drizzle with oil. Cook the asparagus and leeks in batches if needed – they should cover the bottom of the pan in a single layer. Season with sea salt and black pepper and cook until lightly coloured on all sides. Remove to a bowl and rip over half the herbs. Add a squeeze of lemon juice. Leave to one side while you cook the scallops.

Get the same pan nice and hot, score the scallops halfway through in a criss-cross fashion on one side, season them on both sides with some salt, pepper and the five-spice, then drizzle the pan with a few lugs of oil and add the scallops. Fry for a couple of minutes, or until golden, flip them over, add the rest of the herbs and cook for 1 more minute.

While the scallops are cooking, divide the leeks and asparagus between 4 warmed plates. Remove the pan from the heat and add 2 good knobs of butter and the juice of ½ the lemon. Shake the pan about, then put 3 scallops and a little bit of juice on to each plate. Serve immediately and get stuck in.

CALORIES	FAT	SAT FAT	PROTEIN	CARBS	SUGAR	SALT	FIBRE
166kcal	7.6g	3.3g	18.3g	6.6g	3.6g	0.3g	0g

Wicked Baked Sardines

My inspiration for this dish came from the lovely Rose Gray at the River Café, where she would do fantastic things with sardines. The great thing about these is that you can have two or three for a snack, or just one as an appetizer. Feel free to improvise around the herb and breadcrumb story. Scrumptious, mate.

PS Get your fishmonger to prepare the fillets for you.

SERVES 4

1 small bulb of fennel, with herby tops • 1 stale ciabatta loaf, crusts removed • 1 handful of pine nuts, lightly toasted • 1 bunch of fresh marjoram, leaves picked • olive oil • 8 slices of pancetta or dry-cured smoked bacon • 8 fresh sardines, scaled, gutted, filleted • 8 fresh rosemary twigs or cocktail sticks

Remove the herby tops and stalk from the fennel. Put the herby tops to one side and discard the stalks. Halve the fennel bulb, and finely chop. Whiz the ciabatta to coarse breadcrumbs in a food processor or finely chop with a knife, and put the crumbs into a bowl with the fennel, pine nuts and marjoram. Season well with sea salt and black pepper and mix in 4 or 5 tablespoons of oil.

Preheat the oven to 220°C/425°F/gas 7. On a clean board, lay out 1 slice of pancetta. Place a sardine fillet, skin-side down, across it at right angles. Sprinkle the sardine with some of the breadcrumb mix, place another sardine fillet, skin side up, on top of it, sprinkle with a little more breadcrumb mix, then tightly wrap the pancetta around it and spike with a rosemary twig or cocktail stick. Repeat until you have 8 small sardine sandwiches. Lay them on oiled greaseproof paper in a roasting tray and roast at the top of the preheated oven for 8 minutes, or until the bacon and breadcrumbs are crisp.

Serve with rocket salad, a wedge of lemon, and sprinkle over the herby fennel tops. And lads, if you can't pull the birds with that, you might as well give up now!

CALORIES	FAT	SAT FAT	PROTEIN	CARBS	SUGAR	SALT	FIBRE
511kcal	28.4g	6g	26.5g	29.3g	3g	1.5g	2.9g

Roasted Red Mullet
Stuffed with Breadcrumbs, Sun-dried Tomatoes, Olives, Pine Nuts & Marjoram

A lovely way of livening up what is really a simple piece of roasted fish. It might be worth you cooking an extra fish so that the next day you can remove it from the bone, tear it up, toss it with some green leaves, oil and lemon and serve on some toasted bruschetta. A nice little starter.

SERVES 4

½ a ciabatta loaf • 1 large handful of olives, stone in •
1 large handful of sun-dried tomatoes, in oil, chopped •
1 large handful of pine nuts • 1 bunch of fresh marjoram or
basil, leaves picked • olive oil • 4 x 225g whole red mullet,
scaled, gutted, scored

Preheat your oven to 200°C/400°F/gas 6. Remove the crusts from the ciabatta and either whiz the bread up in a food processor until you have small but coarse breadcrumbs, or use a knife to chop the bread finely. Squash the olives, remove the stones and chop. Put the bread into a bowl with the sun-dried tomatoes, olives, pine nuts and marjoram and mix together, loosening with a couple of lugs of oil.

Season the fish inside and out with sea salt and black pepper and place on an oiled baking tray or pan. Stuff the insides with the bread mixture, pushing some into the scored slits and sprinkling any extra around the fish. Roast at the top of the oven for around 20 minutes, or until the fish is cooked. Serve, ideally, with a crisp green salad – I normally sprinkle the excess breadcrumbs over the salad as well for added crunch (how orgasmic is that?!).

CALORIES	FAT	SAT FAT	PROTEIN	CARBS	SUGAR	SALT	FIBRE
444kcal	20g	1.4g	46.9g	20.1g	2.3g	1.8g	1.6g

NICE BIT OF MEAT… At the weekend it's definitely worth getting in some really nice organic meat and spoiling yourself, family and friends. When I buy meat I'm always tempted to buy a little more than I need, so I can use the scrumptious leftovers to make delicious sandwiches, stews, soups or things like shepherd's pie. This chapter contains some of my absolute favourite meat dishes, with inspiration from all around the world. There's nothing better than having a load of mates round for dinner and serving up the tastiest roast. Have a little flick through and see what takes your fancy – there are some really simple recipes as well as some quite indulgent ones, too.

Slow-roasted Duck
with Sage, Ginger & Rhubarb Sauce

This is one of the best duck recipes I've ever had. Slow-roasting means the skin goes really crispy and you cook out loads of fat (which you can keep in the fridge or freezer for roasting your potatoes in the future), and the meat becomes tender, sticky and fantastically rich.

SERVES 4

2 x 1.5kg whole Gresham, Aylesbury or mallard ducks •
250g ginger, peeled • 2 long sticks of baby rhubarb, trimmed •
1 bunch of fresh sage, leaves picked and roughly chopped •
1 bulb of garlic, cloves removed and halved • 2 red onions,
peeled and finely sliced • 2 wineglasses Marsala or Vin Santo •
300ml quality vegetable, chicken or duck stock • olive oil

Preheat the oven to 180°C/350°F/gas 4. Season the ducks generously inside and out with sea salt and black pepper. Coarsely grate half the ginger and rhubarb. Mix this in a bowl with half the sage and all the garlic and onion, and stuff inside the cavity of the ducks. Place them on a tray and roast in the oven for 1 hour, then turn the temperature down to 150°C/300°F/gas 2 and cook for 1 hour 30 minutes, or until crisp and tender. During this time, you'll need to drain the fat maybe 3 times into a bowl – it will separate into clear fat which you can keep for roasting.

Once cooked, allow the ducks to rest on a warmed plate while you make the sauce. Drain off any remaining fat from the roasting tray. Pull out all the stuffing and any juices from the inside of the ducks into the roasting tray. Heat the tray on a low heat, add the Marsala and loosen all the sticky goodness from the bottom – this may flame, so mind your eyebrows! Add the stock and reduce to a good taste and consistency, then pass through a coarse sieve. With a knife you can easily remove the breasts from the ducks and, using your hands, remove the thighs. Divide between plates. To finish, finely slice the remaining ginger and fry off in a little hot oil in a non-stick frying pan. As it begins to colour, add the rest of the rhubarb, finely sliced, and finish with the rest of the sage until crisp. Sprinkle this over the duck and drizzle with the tasty sauce.

CALORIES	FAT	SAT FAT	PROTEIN	CARBS	SUGAR	SALT	FIBRE
628kcal	39.7g	11.8g	37.6g	13.4g	10.2g	0.6g	1.4g

Pot-roasted Pork in White Wine with Garlic, Fennel & Rosemary

This pork recipe takes me about 5 minutes to prepare and get in the oven, so it's nice and quick as well as being unbelievably light, fresh and tasty. Also, pot-roasting the pork as opposed to straight roasting gives you a lovely natural sauce made with the meat juices and the wine. Seriously tasty!

SERVES 6

1 x 1.5kg loin of pork, bone out, skin off • 1 tablespoon fennel seeds • 2–3 large knobs of unsalted butter • olive oil • 8 cloves of garlic • ½ a bunch of fresh rosemary, leaves picked • 4 fresh bay leaves • 1 fennel bulb, sliced • ½ a bottle of Chardonnay

Preheat the oven to 200°C/400°F/gas 6. With 2 or 3 bits of string, tie up the pork loin (see pictures opposite) – do this any way you like. It doesn't have to be fussy, you just want to keep the meat in a snug shape while it's cooking. Season generously with sea salt and black pepper, then roll the meat in the fennel seeds until covered. In a casserole pan or roasting tray, fry the meat for a couple of minutes in half the butter and a little oil, until nice and golden.

Throw in the unpeeled garlic, herbs, fennel and wine, then cover the tray loosely with some wet greaseproof paper and place in the oven for 1 hour 15 minutes. As the pork loin is off the bone it cooks very quickly. Remove from the oven and allow the meat to rest on a plate. Then, without using any more heat, finish off the sauce in the pan, scraping any goodness off the bottom and adding the rest of the butter. Remove any large bits of rosemary if you prefer – but I like to keep it nice and rustic. Taste and correct the seasoning and squash open a couple of the garlic cloves – when cooked they go nice and sweet and add a lovely taste to the sauce.

CALORIES	FAT	SAT FAT	PROTEIN	CARBS	SUGAR	SALT	FIBRE
569kcal	33.5g	12.8g	53.6g	2.9g	1.5g	0.5g	0.2g

Superb Marinated Pork Fillet Roasted on Rhubarb

This dish always surprises people when I serve it to them. The pork fillet doesn't take long to cook, and by roasting it on the rhubarb you'll get fantastic flavours and a superb juice. An excellent accompaniment to the rich meat, just like apple sauce.

SERVES 4

1 bunch of fresh sage, leaves picked • 2 cloves of garlic, peeled
• olive oil • 2 pork fillets, trimmed • 10 slices of prosciutto or
Parma ham • 12 long sticks of baby rhubarb, trimmed

Bash half the sage in a pestle and mortar or use a metal bowl with a rolling pin. Add the garlic and smash. Muddle in 5 tablespoons of oil, then rub the mixture all over the pork and marinate for 1 hour, if possible (I've been known to cook the meat straight away, so it's not the end of the world if you don't have time).

Preheat the oven to 220°C/425°F/gas 7. Lightly season the pork with sea salt and black pepper and drape 5 slices of prosciutto over each fillet – any excess marinade can be rubbed on to this as well. Cut the rhubarb into finger-sized pieces and place in an appropriately-sized roasting tray (preferably not aluminium, as it will taint the rhubarb). Place the pork on top of the rhubarb, almost tucking it into bed! Sprinkle over the rest of the sage leaves and drizzle with oil. Get yourself a piece of greaseproof paper, wet it and scrunch it up, then lay it over the meat and tuck it in round the sides. Cook in the oven for 15 minutes, then remove the paper and cook for an extra 15 minutes, or until golden and cooked through.

Remove from the oven and leave to rest for about 5 minutes. I slice the meat at an angle, giving each person half a fillet each. Pour any juice that comes out of the meat back into the roasting tray. Serve the meat with the rhubarb, the lovely juices from the tray and roast potatoes.

CALORIES	FAT	SAT FAT	PROTEIN	CARBS	SUGAR	SALT	FIBRE
420kcal	24.8g	5.4g	47.2g	2.2g	1g	1g	1.7g

Flour & Water Crust Chicken

This is a great dish to serve up to friends – they'll wonder if you've gone a bit mad when you produce what looks like a huge lump of pastry and put it in the middle of the table! It's a great way to cook chicken – the meat steams inside the pastry crust and becomes incredibly tender. I've used nice small spring chickens, or poussins, in this recipe but it's just as easy to use one 2kg bird and roast it for 2 hours instead. PS You don't eat the pastry!

SERVES 4

900g plain flour • 2 fat lemons • 1 bunch of fresh sage, leaves picked • ½ a bunch of fresh thyme, leaves picked • 8 cloves of garlic, peeled • olive oil • 4 whole spring chickens

Put the flour into a large bowl, and mix in around 500ml of water, bit by bit, until you have a dough that is pliable and elastic and not too sticky. Cover and put to one side while you prepare the chickens.

Using a speed-peeler, remove the peel from 1 of the lemons and bash up with the sage, thyme and garlic in a pestle and mortar, or use a metal bowl and a rolling pin. Muddle in 8 tablespoons of oil, then season well with sea salt and black pepper. This flavourful marinade is great with just about all kinds of meat. Roll up your sleeves and rub the marinade all over the chickens as well as inside the cavity. Slice the remaining lemon and stick a slice or two inside the cavity of each chicken.

Preheat the oven to 220°C/425°F/gas 7. Get the dough mix, divide it into 4 pieces, and roll each one out to about ½cm thick. Now mould a piece of dough around each of the chickens so that you have 4 airtight parcels. Leave for 5 minutes, then bake in the oven for 1 hour – the crust will harden during cooking, steaming and protecting the chicken while keeping all the lovely juices inside, which will give you a fantastic homemade gravy.

Let the chickens rest for 15 minutes after baking, then bring them to the table and, for a bit of drama, crack open each crust in front of your guests. You'll unleash a wicked aroma, steam, the lot, so waft it around a bit. Very impressive stuff. Delicious served simply with some potatoes and greens.

CALORIES	FAT	SAT FAT	PROTEIN	CARBS	SUGAR	SALT	FIBRE
656kcal	49.5g	10.2g	49.8g	3.1g	0.5g	1.4g	0.7g

Pot-roasted Chicken
with Sweet & Sour Sauce

This is a fantastic but slightly tacky-sounding roast chicken dish. I have to keep reinventing chicken dishes, as Jools makes me cook chicken every Sunday. It starts to do my head in a bit, but this is one of my latest little winners that always puts a smile on her funny little face.

SERVES 6

1 x 2kg whole chicken • 1 bunch of fresh flat-leaf parsley, leaves picked and roughly chopped • 4 x 5cm pieces of ginger, grated with skin left on • 2 red peppers, halved and deseeded • 2 yellow peppers, halved and deseeded • 4 red onions, peeled • 2 fresh red chillies, halved • 1 ripe pineapple, peeled, quartered and chopped • 1 teaspoon fennel seeds, crushed • olive oil • 2 tablespoons sugar • 6 tablespoons balsamic vinegar

Preheat the oven to 190°C/375°F/gas 5. Season the chicken generously inside and out with sea salt and black pepper and stuff the cavity with the parsley and ginger. Cut the peppers and red onions into quarters and put them into a cold casserole pan. Add the chillies, pineapple and crushed fennel seeds. Drizzle with 3 good lugs of oil, sprinkle with salt and pepper, and toss until well-coated. Place the chicken on top, pat it with a little oil and cook in the middle of the oven for 1 hour 30 minutes – the chicken is ready when the juices run clear.

Once cooked, drain the chicken juices over the pan. Remove the chicken to a plate with half the vegetables and pineapple, and allow to rest for 5 minutes while you make the sauce. Put the remaining vegetables and pineapple from the pan into a food processor with the sugar and balsamic vinegar, taste and correct the seasoning. Blend to make a lovely sauce – add a little boiling water to loosen, if needed. You could pass it through a coarse sieve to make it even smoother, but I don't. Taste and correct the seasoning, if needed.

To be honest, I can't think of anything better to serve the chicken with than some simple stir-fried noodles or some steamed or boiled rice. Just put the chicken and the veg in the middle of the table and tuck in.

CALORIES	FAT	SAT FAT	PROTEIN	CARBS	SUGAR	SALT	FIBRE
439kcal	19.6g	4g	35.5g	31.8g	29.3g	0.4g	4.7g

Chicken in Salt
with Fennel, Thyme & Lemon

Possibly the maddest recipe in the world and, before you think it, this is not over-salty. It's probably one of the most luxurious chicken dishes you can have. Your friends will think you've completely lost it when you come out to the table with a block of salt and a pickaxe (joke).

SERVES 6

3kg coarse rock salt • 8 heaped tablespoons fennel seeds, cracked • 2 large eggs, beaten • 2 lemons • 1 tablespoon peppercorns • 1 bunch of fresh thyme • olive oil • 1 x 2kg whole chicken • 1 bunch of fresh flat-leaf parsley, ripped • 8 cloves of garlic

Preheat the oven to 200°C/400°F/gas 6. Put all the salt into a bowl with the fennel seeds, eggs, lemon juice (keep the skins), peppercorns and a wineglass of water, then mix together. Strip the thyme leaves into a pestle and mortar, bash to a paste, then muddle in a couple of good lugs of oil. Rub all over the chicken, pushing any excess inside the cavity along with the parsley, unpeeled garlic cloves and squeezed lemon halves – the idea here is to tightly pack the cavity so it bulges and no salt can get in.

Get 4 long pieces of tin foil and put them on top of each other to make a sheet around 1 metre square. Lay on a third of the salt, making it about 2cm thick. Put the chicken on top, then pack the rest of the salt around it. Because the salt is slightly wet it should stick to the chicken – make sure that the chicken's skin hasn't been pierced. Carefully fold up the sides of the foil and scrunch it at the top. You can rip off any excess – basically the foil is there to hold the salt together until it hardens.

Roast the chicken in the oven for 2 hours, then remove and allow to rest for 15 minutes. Take it to the table with one or two really nice salads, some bread and a bottle of white wine. Rip open the foil and crack the salt crust – it will fall apart easily and reveal the fantastic-smelling chicken. Pull the skin away and tear the meat from the thighs and the breast – absolutely pukka. Gorgeous served with horseradish mixed with crème fraîche or homemade basil mayonnaise.

CALORIES	FAT	SAT FAT	PROTEIN	CARBS	SUGAR	SALT	FIBRE
430kcal	24.9g	6.7g	51.6g	0.1g	0g	1.4g	0.1g

Chicken in Milk

A slightly odd but really fantastic combination which must be tried.

SERVES 4

1 x 1.5kg whole chicken • 100g unsalted butter • olive oil •
½ a cinnamon stick • 1 bunch of fresh sage, leaves picked •
2 lemons • 10 cloves of garlic • 550ml milk

Preheat the oven to 190°C/375°F/gas 5, and find a snug-fitting pot for the chicken. Season the chicken generously with sea salt and black pepper, and fry it in the butter and a little oil, turning regularly to get an even colour all over. Remove from the heat, put the chicken on a plate, and throw away the oil and butter left in the pot. This will leave you with tasty sticky goodness at the bottom of the pan which will give you a lovely caramelly flavour later on.

Put the chicken back in the pot with the rest of the ingredients (speed-peel the lemon zest and leave the garlic cloves unpeeled), and cook in the preheated oven for 1 hour 30 minutes, basting with the cooking juice when you remember. The lemon zest will sort of split the milk, making a sauce which is absolutely fantastic.

To serve, pull the meat off the bones and divide between plates. Spoon over plenty of juice and the little curds. Delicious served with wilted spinach or greens and some mashed potato.

CALORIES	FAT	SAT FAT	PROTEIN	CARBS	SUGAR	SALT	FIBRE
533kcal	35.7g	15.6g	44.7g	9.2g	6.9g	1g	0.5g

My Old Man's Superb Chicken

SERVES 4

170g mushrooms, any combination • olive oil • 1 or 2 cloves
of garlic, peeled and finely chopped • 1 bunch of fresh
flat-leaf parsley, leaves picked and chopped • 4 chicken breasts,
skin off • plain flour, for dusting • 320g puff pastry • 1 large
egg, beaten • 2 heaped tablespoons wholegrain mustard •
1 large wineglass of white wine • 140ml double cream •
optional: extra virgin olive oil

Preheat the oven to 200°C/400°F/gas 6. Chop the mushrooms – half rough and half fine. Put a couple of lugs of olive oil into a hot pan and slowly fry the garlic with the mushrooms for about 10 minutes. Season to taste with sea salt and black pepper and stir in the chopped parsley. Allow to cool. Pull back the chicken fillet on the breast and, keeping it intact, score into the breast and stuff the chicken with the cooled mushrooms (see pictures opposite).

On a clean, flour-dusted surface, roll the pastry out to around 45cm in length, 20cm wide. Slice into 4 pieces, lengthways, and wrap around each chicken breast (see pictures below). Brush the pastry with a little beaten egg, and cook in the oven for 35 minutes, or until golden and cooked through. While the chicken is cooking, put the mustard and white wine into a hot pan and allow to reduce until you've cooked away the alcohol smell. Add the cream and simmer until the sauce coats the back of a spoon, then remove from the heat and season to taste. Slice each chicken breast into 3 and serve with a bit of sauce and a little drizzle of extra virgin olive oil, if you like. Bloomin' gorgeous.

CALORIES	FAT	SAT FAT	PROTEIN	CARBS	SUGAR	SALT	FIBRE
423kcal	26.5g	11.2g	22.8g	19.2g	1.9g	1.2g	1.8g

Pan-roasted Guinea Fowl
with Pomegranate & Spinach

SERVES 2

1 x 1kg guinea fowl, chicken or pheasant • 100g ricotta cheese • ½ a bunch of fresh thyme, leaves picked and chopped • olive oil • 1 knob of unsalted butter • 1 clove of garlic, peeled and finely sliced • ½ a wineglass of white wine • 1 pomegranate, seeds removed, skin and yellow pith discarded • 2 large handfuls of baby spinach

Remove the drumsticks, thighs and breasts from the bird (see pictures below) or ask your butcher to do this for you. In a small bowl, beat the ricotta and thyme together. Season lightly with sea salt and black pepper. Using two fingers, delicately part the skin from the breast and the skin from the drumsticks and thighs. With a teaspoon, insert the ricotta mix into these gaps, then pull the skin down to cover.

Preheat the oven to 220°C/425°F/gas 7. Season the bird, then drizzle an ovenproof pan with a little oil and fry the drumsticks and thighs for 5 minutes, or until golden and crisp. Add the breasts, skin-side up, with a large knob of butter, the garlic and the wine. Place at the top of the oven and cook for 25 minutes, then add the pomegranate seeds and cook for an extra 5 minutes, by which time your thigh meat will be cooked all the way through and the skin will be crispy. Take the pan out of the oven and place back on the hob. Add the spinach and let it wilt. You will have a great homemade sauce at the bottom of the pan. Taste and check the seasoning – it should be fine – then serve a breast, thigh and drumstick on each plate with the spinach and pomegranates in and around it. Drizzle over the homemade sauce and serve with some boiled potatoes.

CALORIES	FAT	SAT FAT	PROTEIN	CARBS	SUGAR	SALT	FIBRE
629kcal	38.2g	13.4g	58.4g	5.5g	4.3g	1.1g	1.1g

Japanese Rolled Pork
with Plums, Coriander, Soy Sauce & Spring Onions

This is a fantastic appetizer that I had in Japan. With there being no fat on the pork and it being steamed, it's a very clean and tasty dish.

SERVES 4

10 plums • 2 tablespoons olive oil • 2 star anise •
10cm piece of ginger, peeled and finely grated • 2 cloves •
2 heaped tablespoons muscovado sugar • 600g pork loin •
½ a bunch of fresh coriander, leaves picked and chopped •
spring onions • low-salt soy sauce

Run a knife around the plums, then twist and remove the stones. Cut the halves into 1cm dice. Drizzle 2 tablespoons of oil into a pan and fry the star anise, ginger and cloves for 1 minute. Add the plums and sugar with a couple of tablespoons of water, place a lid on, and simmer slowly for about 20 minutes, or until chunky and pulpy. Allow to cool in the fridge.

Trim all the fat and sinews from the pork so that you're left with just lean eye meat. Cut into ½cm slices and one by one bash the slices between 2 pieces of greaseproof, using something flat and heavy like the base of a heavy pan, a meat hammer or a cleaver. Try to retain the pork's shape. When each piece is around the thickness of two beer mats, carefully peel the meat away from the paper in one piece. Do this with all the meat and lay it out on a tray.

Season the plum sauce with sea salt and black pepper, then stir in half the coriander. Spread 1 tablespoon of the sauce in the middle of each slice of pork so that the sauce covers about three-quarters of each slice, then roll each one up like a Swiss roll. Put the rolls into a bamboo steamer (if you have one) or a normal steamer, or even use a colander covered in tin foil. Place the steamer over simmering water and steam for 10 to 15 minutes, or until the meat is just cooked. Remove from the steamer and serve the pork rolls on a bed of finely sliced spring onions, sprinkled with the rest of the coriander and doused with lots of soy sauce.

CALORIES	FAT	SAT FAT	PROTEIN	CARBS	SUGAR	SALT	FIBRE
398kcal	14.6g	3.6g	45.8g	22.7g	21.6g	1.6g	0.2g

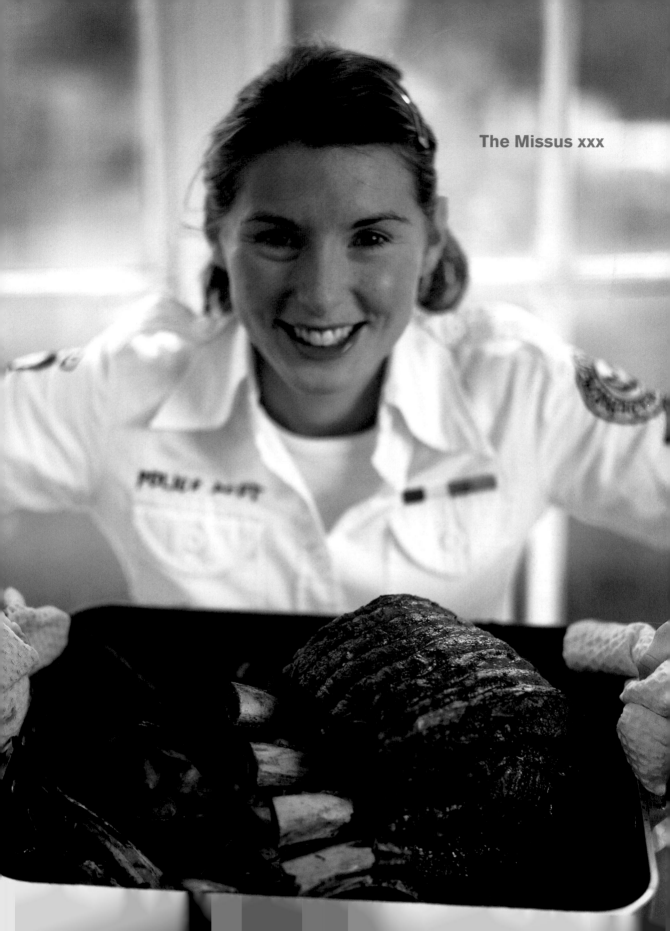

The Missus xxx

Superb Roast Beef, Best Spuds & Huge Yorkies

SERVES 8

1 x 2.5kg fore-rib, wing-rib or sirloin of beef,
French-trimmed • olive oil • 3 red onions, halved •
3kg potatoes, peeled and roughly chopped • 4 large parsnips,
peeled and quartered • 3 fresh rosemary twigs • 4 cloves of
garlic, peeled • 10cm piece of ginger, peeled and diced •
plain flour • ½ a bottle of robust red wine

Roasting is easy, but timing is important. Before you start, get all the veg prepped and have the Yorkshire pudding batter made (see page 25). With this done, you can get the Yorkshires and greens on while the beef is resting out of the oven.

Preheat the oven to 230°C/450°F/gas 8, and heat a large roasting tray on the hob. Rub the beef generously with sea salt, then add a little olive oil to the tray and lightly colour the meat on all sides for a couple of minutes. Lay the onions in the tray with the beef on top of them, then cook into the oven for a total of 1 hour 30 minutes. While the beef is starting, parboil the potatoes in boiling salted water for around 10 minutes, then drain. Toss them about in the colander to chuff them up – this will make them really crispy.

After 30 minutes, take the tray out of the oven and toss in the potatoes, parsnips and rosemary. With a garlic press or grater, squeeze or grate the garlic and ginger over everything in the tray. Shake the tray and whack it back into the oven for the final hour. Remove the potatoes and parsnips to a dish to keep warm, place the beef on a plate, covered with tin foil, to rest, and get the greens and Yorkshire puddings on. Preheat a Yorkshire pudding tray with 1cm of oil in each section. After 10 minutes, divide the batter into the tray. Cook for around 30 minutes, or until crisp – don't open the oven door before then or they won't rise.

Remove most of the fat from the roasting tray and you should be left with caramelized onions and sticky beef goodness. Add 1 teaspoon of flour to the tray and mash everything together. Heat the tray on the hob and when hot, add the red wine. Simmer for 5 to 10 minutes, or until your gravy is really tasty and coats the back of a spoon, stirring every couple of minutes. Add any juice from the beef and feel free to add some water or stock to loosen the gravy, if you like. Pour through a coarse sieve, pushing it through with a spoon, and serve in a warmed gravy jug.

CALORIES	FAT	SAT FAT	PROTEIN	CARBS	SUGAR	SALT	FIBRE
760kcal	26.8g	11.6g	44.5g	81.2g	11.2g	1.1g	11.2g

THESE VALUES EXCLUDE THE YORKSHIRE PUDDINGS (SEE PAGE 25)

PS Serve up the Yorkies and veg with some horseradish sauce and carve the beef at the table. Just so you know, beef needs 30 minutes per kilo to cook, plus an extra 20 minutes at the end, no matter how big it is. This will cook it medium, so give it a bit more or less depending on your preference.

Medallions of Beef
with Morels & Marsala & Crème Fraîche Sauce

I always think of this as being quite a luxurious dinner. But even though it uses dried morels and medallions of beef, which are never cheap, it's a real quickie to make. Medallions of beef are basically 1cm thick slices of beef fillet that are normally grilled or fried. You can get your butcher to prep these for you, or cut a fillet steak in half and flatten it out slightly yourself.

SERVES 4

2 handfuls of dried morels • 1 bunch of fresh thyme, leaves picked • 8 x 85g beef fillet medallions • 2 shallots, peeled and finely chopped • 1 clove of garlic, peeled and finely chopped • 1 wineglass of Marsala • 4 tablespoons crème fraîche

Put the dried morels into a small bowl and cover with boiling water. Finely chop half the thyme leaves and sprinkle over the medallions with a little oil. Rub the thyme and oil into the meat and allow to sit for 10 minutes.

Get a large, non-stick frying pan hot, season the steaks on both sides with sea salt and black pepper, and sear them for just over 2 minutes on each side – they will go slightly golden and will be cooked medium by this time, which is the way I like them. Feel free to cook for longer, or less time, to your liking. Remove the meat to a plate and allow to rest for 4 or 5 minutes while you make the sauce.

Turn down the heat, add a little extra oil to the pan, and throw in the shallots, garlic and remaining thyme. After 1 minute, strain the morels and add them – I like to leave three-quarters of them whole and finely chop the rest. Add the Marsala – this may flame up in the pan for about 20 seconds, which is fine, so don't be shocked. It will smell fantastic. Add the crème fraîche and any juices that have come out of the meat. Season to taste. The sauce should coat the back of a spoon – loosen it with water if it gets too thick. Give each person 2 medallions, pour the sauce over, and serve with something nice and stodgy like mashed potato, or the smashed celeriac on page 216. Also great with the braised greens on page 211.

PS If you have thyme growing on your windowsill, snip off some tender leaves and sprinkle over just before serving. A delicious thyme-fest!

CALORIES	FAT	SAT FAT	PROTEIN	CARBS	SUGAR	SALT	FIBRE
378kcal	19.4g	9.6g	35.9g	6.7g	4.7g	0.7g	1.4g

Traybaked Lamb
with Aubergines, Tomatoes, Olives, Garlic & Mint Oil

SERVES 6

2 x 6-rib racks of lamb, French-trimmed • 2 firm aubergines •
8 ripe plum tomatoes • olive oil • 8 cloves of garlic • dried
oregano • optional: a few sprigs of fresh basil or marjoram •
1 handful of olives, stone in • 1 big bunch of fresh mint • pinch
of sugar • good red wine vinegar • extra virgin olive oil

Preheat the oven to 200°C/400°F/gas 6. Criss-cross the fat on the lamb – this will help it render and become nice and crisp. Place to one side.

Slice the aubergines widthways into 2.5cm thick pieces and slice the tomatoes in half. Lightly brush the aubergine slices all over with olive oil, then fry on both sides in a non-stick pan to give them just a little colour. Remove the aubergines from the pan and place on one side of a clean roasting tray. Put the halved tomatoes and whole unpeeled garlic cloves beside them and sprinkle with a little oregano and sea salt and black pepper. You could always rip a little fresh basil or marjoram over the tomatoes as well.

Season the lamb and fry in your non-stick pan until lightly golden on all sides. Drizzle with a little olive oil, then place the lamb skin side up next to the aubergines and tomatoes and bake in the oven for 30 minutes to retain a little pinkness – but you can always cook it to suit your taste. Squash the olives, remove the stones and add to the roasting tray for the last 5 minutes so they warm through. Remove from the oven and allow the lamb to rest for 5 minutes.

Now make some fantastic mint oil. Put the mint into a pestle and mortar or a blender with a pinch each of salt and sugar, and blitz up until smooth. Add a couple of tablespoons of good red wine vinegar and loosen with 6 tablespoons of extra virgin olive oil. Season to taste and tweak with a little more vinegar, if needed. This is a fantastic sauce that is great drizzled over the veg and lamb. I like to cut my lamb in half between the ribs and then divide each half into 3 cutlets.

PS When you buy your racks of lamb, ask your butcher to 'French-trim' them, which means that all the bones are scraped clean – this looks nice and pretty and it cooks easier as well.

CALORIES	FAT	SAT FAT	PROTEIN	CARBS	SUGAR	SALT	FIBRE
526kcal	41.2g	15.4g	33g	6.1g	4.4g	1.3g	2.9g

. . . AND LOADS OF VEG People are always wondering how to completely turn around their day-to-day cooking to make things more exciting. Or maybe even a bit healthier. Here's your answer – a stonking little vegetable section. Even though I'm becoming slightly more eclectic in my old age, the Mediterranean use of vegetables and flavourings is still my favourite. My recipes in this vegetable chapter are really superb. They're quite modern British in style, with things like Minty Mushy Peas, Smashed Celeriac and World's Best Baked Onions.

When at all possible, try using some more unusual vegetables because if we don't try them the shops won't keep stocking them. Over the last couple of years there's been a revolution of weekend farmers' markets. Please try to support these people as their true passion for growing and supplying excellent produce can teach us all something.

Minty Mushy Peas

This is a fantastic recipe which is so quick and so simple and uses our reliable friends the frozen peas, which work really well here. Great with fish, meat or even as a vegetarian dish with a big dollop of butter on top.

SERVES 4–6

2 medium potatoes, peeled and finely diced •
1kg frozen peas • 1 bunch of fresh mint, leaves picked •
3 large knobs of unsalted butter

Cook the potatoes in boiling salted water until nearly tender. Add the peas to the pan, then after 2 minutes of boiling add the mint. After another minute, drain everything into a colander. Leave for 1 minute to steam, then put everything back into the pan and mash with a potato masher. You can do this in a food processor as well – just pulse it until smooth. Whether mashing or pulsing, when it's done add the butter and season very carefully to taste with sea salt and black pepper.

CALORIES	FAT	SAT FAT	PROTEIN	CARBS	SUGAR	SALT	FIBRE
283kcal	8g		14.8g	40.1g	14.9g	0.4g	14.5g

World's Best Baked Onions

I've found it. The very best onion recipe – it's smashing, pukka, the absolute dog's kahunas! I love it served with cod but it's also great with roast chicken. Try it!

SERVES 4

4 tennis-ball sized onions, peeled • olive oil • 2 cloves of garlic, peeled and finely chopped • 4 twigs of fresh rosemary, lower leaves picked and chopped • 8 tablespoons double cream • a couple of handfuls of freshly grated Parmesan cheese • 4 slices of pancetta or dry-cured smoked streaky bacon

Boil the onions in plenty of water for 15 minutes, or until slightly tender. Remove from the pan and allow to cool. Then, with a sharp knife, remove the top 2.5cm of each onion, finely chop and keep to one side. If needed, slightly trim the stalk end of the onions so that they will sit flat on a roasting tray. Cut about 1 heaped tablespoon out from the inside of each onion, keeping the outside intact. Finely chop and add to the rest of the chopped onion.

Preheat the oven to 200°C/400°F/gas 6. Drizzle a little olive oil into a hot frying pan and add the garlic, the chopped onions and just a little chopped rosemary. Fry for 2 minutes, or until softened, then turn the heat down, add the cream and remove from the heat. Stir in the Parmesan and season with sea salt and black pepper.

I like to wrap a nice slice of pancetta around the middle of each onion and just spike it in place with a sharpened twig of rosemary or half a cocktail stick. The rosemary and pancetta will make the onion taste lovely as it cooks. Place the onions on a roasting tray and spoon some of the chopped onion mixture inside each one. Bake in the oven for 25 minutes, or until tender, depending on the size of the onions. It's cool to experiment with different cheeses, so give it a bash.

CALORIES	FAT	SAT FAT	PROTEIN	CARBS	SUGAR	SALT	FIBRE
263kcal	20.3g	11.8g	5.1g	16g	11.8g	0.5g	4.6g

Baked Peppers
with Cherry Vine Tomatoes, Basil & Marjoram

SERVES 4

2 peppers, red or yellow • 20 ripe cherry tomatoes • 1 bunch
of fresh marjoram and basil • 2 cloves of garlic, peeled and
sliced • optional: anchovy fillets, in oil • olive oil •
optional: herb vinegar

Preheat the oven to 200°C/400°F/gas 6. Cut the peppers in half and remove the seeds. Place in an oiled baking dish and lightly season with sea salt and black pepper. Prick the cherry tomatoes with a knife and place in boiling water for around 30 to 60 seconds, or until the skins can be easily and quickly pinched off. Feel free to run cold water over them before peeling. Once peeled, place the tomatoes in the peppers. Stuff in the herbs and sliced garlic, then season. You could drape over some anchovies instead of using seasoning at this point. Drizzle with oil. Cook in the oven for 15 minutes lightly covered with tin foil, then around 30 minutes without. A little splash of herb vinegar on each pepper is a real joy.

CALORIES	FAT	SAT FAT	PROTEIN	CARBS	SUGAR	SALT	FIBRE
34kcal	1.8g	0.3g	0.8g	3.8g	3.3g	0.3g	1.7g

Braised Greens

This is a really simple and tasty way to make greens less boring. Also, having a mixture of greens makes things much more appealing. I've used three types of greens, including rocket, which is always thought of as a salad leaf. Cicoria is a slightly bitter-tasting green leaf which is excellent for braising. If you can't get hold of it, try substituting any other type of green, like spinach, cabbage, cavolo nero, Chinese leaf, beet leaves, sprouting broccoli – whatever you fancy.

SERVES 4

2 large handfuls of Swiss chard • 2 large handfuls of cicoria or
any of the leaves mentioned above • olive oil • 2 large cloves of
garlic, peeled and finely sliced • 2 large handfuls of rocket •
½ a lemon

Half-fill a large pot with salted water, bring to the boil and add the Swiss chard and cicoria. Cook for 2 or 3 minutes, or until the greens are tender, or al dente, then drain in a colander. To the empty pan, add 4 large lugs of oil and the garlic. Fry the garlic until lightly coloured, then throw in the cooked cicoria and chard. Season with sea salt and black pepper and stir around to coat in all the lovely flavoured oil. After 1 minute, remove from the heat, add the rocket and squeeze in the lemon juice. Stir once more, check the seasoning again, and serve immediately. Great with grilled meats or scallops, or even served cold on an antipasti plate.

CALORIES	FAT	SAT FAT	PROTEIN	CARBS	SUGAR	SALT	FIBRE
194kcal	20.3g	2.9g	1.3g	1.6g	0.5g	0.4g	1g

Baked New Potatoes
with Sea Salt & Rosemary

SERVES 6

1.2kg Jersey Royals • 1 tablespoon olive oil • 2 sprigs of fresh
rosemary, leaves picked and bashed

Preheat the oven to 220°C/425°F/gas 7. Scrub the potatoes, parboil in boiling
salted water until almost tender, then drain. Drizzle with 1 tablespoon of oil and roll
in 1 tablespoon of sea salt, a little black pepper and the rosemary. Put the potatoes
into a roasting tray and roast for 25 minutes, or until golden. Alternatively, wrap
them in tin foil and throw them on the barbie for the same amount of time.

CALORIES	FAT	SAT FAT	PROTEIN	CARBS	SUGAR	SALT	FIBRE
680kcal	2.8g	0.5g	3.4g	32.3g	2.6g	0.7g	2g

Dad in the garden

Roasted Asparagus
with Rosemary & Anchovies Wrapped in Pancetta

This is a great vegetable dish, either to have for a starter or as a vegetable with chicken or fish. Having the asparagus tied together looks damn funky and all the ingredients flavour each other as they roast in the oven, which makes them taste sensational. I've used string to tie the bundles together in the picture but it's much better to use a slice of pancetta.

SERVES 4

24 asparagus spears • 4 sprigs of fresh rosemary • 4 anchovy fillets, in oil • 4 good slices of pancetta or dry-cured smoky bacon • ½ a lemon • olive oil • 1 knob of unsalted butter

Preheat the oven to 220°C/425°F/gas 7. Remove the woody ends from the asparagus by bending and snapping them where it clicks naturally. Feel free to boil the asparagus for 1 minute if they're not as tender as they should be. Grab 6 spears of asparagus, sandwich one of the rosemary sprigs and one of the anchovy fillets among the spears, and wrap a slice of pancetta round the middle to hold everything in place. Make 3 more bundles the same way, and put them into a small roasting tray or pan with ½ a lemon. Drizzle with a little oil and roast in the oven for 4 to 5 minutes, or until the pancetta is crispy. Remove from the oven, add the butter, and squeeze over the juice from the roasted lemon. Season with sea salt and black pepper, if needed. This will make a fantastic smoky sauce with your melted anchovies.

CALORIES	FAT	SAT FAT	PROTEIN	CARBS	SUGAR	SALT	FIBRE
94kcal	5.9g	1.5g	6.8g	3.4g	2.9g	0.9g	2.6g

Smashed Celeriac

What a surprisingly simple and comforting veg dish. Unfortunately everyone seems to be completely baffled by celeriac, but it's beautiful in soups or thinly sliced into salads. When roasted it goes sweet and when mixed with potato and mashed it's a complete joy. Trust me, you're going to love it.

SERVES 4

1 celeriac, peeled • olive oil • ½ a bunch of fresh thyme, leaves picked • 2 cloves of garlic, picked and finely chopped • 3–4 tablespoons quality stock

Slice about 1cm off the bottom of the celeriac and roll it on to that flat edge, so it's nice and safe to slice. Slice and dice it all up into 1cm-ish cubes. Don't get your ruler out – they don't have to be perfect. Put a casserole pan on a high heat, add 3 good lugs of oil, then add the celeriac, thyme and garlic, with a little sea salt and black pepper. Stir to coat and fry quite fast for 5 minutes to give it a little colour. Turn the heat down to a simmer, add the stock (or replace with water), place a lid on top and cook for 25 minutes, or until tender. Season carefully to taste and stir with a spoon to smash up the celeriac. Some people like to keep it in cubes, some like to mash it, but I think it looks and tastes much better if you smash it, which is somewhere in the middle. You can serve this with just about any meat you can think of.

CALORIES	FAT	SAT FAT	PROTEIN	CARBS	SUGAR	SALT	FIBRE
153kcal	15.4g	2.2g	1.2g	2.5g	1.4g	0.7g	2.9g

Traybaked Artichokes
with Almonds, Breadcrumbs & Herbs

This veg dish is good for anything – from antipasti to serving with meat or fish.

SERVES 4

8 medium globe artichokes • 1 lemon • 2 cloves of garlic,
peeled and finely chopped • 1 handful of whole almonds, finely
chopped • 2 handfuls of coarse breadcrumbs • 1 bunch of
fresh mint, leaves picked and finely chopped • 1 handful of fresh
flat-leaf parsley, leaves picked and finely chopped • olive oil •
2 wineglasses of white wine

To prepare the artichokes (see pictures opposite), simply trim 5cm below and above the base of the choke. Trim back the artichoke leaves one by one, clicking them off until you get to the lovely paler yellow and more tender leaves. Using a pointed teaspoon, insert it right into the centre of the artichoke flower and slowly turn it to remove the fluffy choke. Have a little peer in and try to remove most of the choke. Rub the artichoke with lemon to stop it discolouring. You'll get the hang of it when you do the rest. You'll be left with 8 whole trimmed artichokes.

Preheat the oven to 200°C/400°F/gas 6. Toss the garlic, almonds, breadcrumbs and herbs into a bowl, season with sea salt and black pepper, and loosen with a little oil. Scrunch together with your hands and stuff this mixture into the middle of each artichoke, really packing it in. You want to fit these snugly side by side in an appropriately-sized baking dish. Sprinkle any excess filling over the top, drizzle generously with oil and pour in the wine. Rip off a big enough piece of greaseproof paper, wet and scrunch it under a tap, then tuck it over the artichokes and round the edges of the dish. Bake in the oven for 30 minutes, then remove the greaseproof paper and bake for a final 10 minutes, or until golden. Serve in the middle of the table with seafood or any white meat.

CALORIES	FAT	SAT FAT	PROTEIN	CARBS	SUGAR	SALT	FIBRE
184kcal	6.9g	0.9g	11.3g	17.3g	8.9g	0.9g	0.4g

Roasted Veg

I love roasted vegetables, and to bump up the veggies on a family dinner there's nothing better than to have 4 to 5 roasted ones all done in the same tray – it's completely effortless and always a treat. There are certain fresh herbs and spices that really go with certain vegetables. Feel free to flavour your veg as you like, but here are my suggestions to give you a bit of a pukka edge to your veg.

All the veg should be cut into similar-sized pieces so that they cook at the same time, tossed separately with their suggested flavourings and seasoned generously. Preheat the oven to 220°C/425°F/gas 7. Place the veg in a large tray next to each other and cover with tin foil. Cook in the oven for 20 minutes, then remove the foil and continue roasting for another 20 to 30 minutes, or until golden and tender. If by any chance one is cooked before another, simply remove from the oven and keep warm in a serving dish.

PS You can cook as many as you like in the same tray, or just one or two. It's up to you.

- halved carrots with a pinch of cumin, fresh rosemary and olive oil
- quartered parsnips with bashed fresh thyme, honey and olive oil
- peeled and sliced celeriac with fresh thyme, rosemary and olive oil
- chunks of squash with crushed coriander seeds, a hint of chilli, fresh oregano and olive oil
- quartered fennel with its own herby tops and olive oil
- whole baby turnips with fresh tarragon, a splash of white wine vinegar and olive oil
- peeled and quartered red onions with fresh sage and olive oil
- scrubbed and halved Jerusalem artichokes with fresh marjoram, rosemary and olive oil

Roasted Fennel
with Cherry Tomatoes, Olives, Garlic & Olive Oil

A great little combo that is tasty and fresh. Any leftovers can be chopped and turned into a sexy little pasta dish, maybe with some ricotta and Parmesan cheese added to it. You could even try putting a couple of chicken breasts on top of the fennel and tomatoes before baking in the oven, to make a tasty dinner.

SERVES 6

2 bulbs of fennel • 24 ripe cherry tomatoes • 1 large handful
of black olives (stone in) • ½ a bunch of fresh thyme, leaves
picked • 2 cloves of garlic, peeled and finely sliced • olive oil •
1 wineglass of white wine, vermouth or Pernod • 2 knobs of
unsalted butter

Remove the top herby stalks from the fennel and slice them finely. Put them into a roasting tray. Cut the fennel bulbs each into 8 wedges. Put them into boiling, salted water and cook for 10 minutes. While the fennel is cooking, preheat the oven to 220°C/425°F/gas 7 and prick the cherry tomatoes with a knife. After 10 minutes remove the fennel with a slotted spoon and add to the roasting tray. Put the tomatoes into the fennel water for 30 to 60 seconds, or until the skins can be easily and quickly pinched off. Add the tomatoes to the roasting tray. Squash the olives and remove the stones, then add to the tray with the thyme and garlic and season with sea salt and black pepper. Drizzle with 2 lugs of oil and mix together. Try to arrange everything neatly so you have one layer. Add the wine and butter, breaking it up over the veg. Bake in the middle of the oven for 30 minutes.

CALORIES	FAT	SAT FAT	PROTEIN	CARBS	SUGAR	SALT	FIBRE
109kcal	6.7g	2.3g	2g	5.3g	4.4g	0.3g	1.1g

Swiss Chard with Cannellini Beans

SERVES 4

2 large handfuls of Swiss chard, trimmed • ½ a bunch of fresh
thyme or summer savory, leaves picked • 2 cloves of garlic,
peeled and thinly sliced • 2 anchovy fillets, in oil • olive oil •
1 x 400g tin of cannellini beans, drained • 1 large knob of
unsalted butter • ½ a lemon

Cook the Swiss chard in boiling salted water until just tender, then drain and
remove to a plate. In the same pot, fry the herbs, garlic and anchovies in a couple
of lugs of oil. Add the cannellini beans, with 1 tablespoon of water to help heat
them through, then after 1 minute add the chard and butter. Toss together and
season to taste with sea salt, black pepper and a little squeeze of lemon juice. Serve
immediately – it's pretty good with anything.

CALORIES	FAT	SAT FAT	PROTEIN	CARBS	SUGAR	SALT	FIBRE
71kcal	6.9g	2g	1g	1.3g	0.2g	0.5g	0.4g

Hamilton Squash

This is a recipe inspired by a one-minute conversation with my mate Johnny Boy Hamilton. He had basically eaten far too much meat in Paris, went for the veggie option one night and was blown away by it. His description used a marrow instead of a squash and some kind of green rice, but anyway, the great thing is I've given this a bash my way and I think it's an absolutely fantastic recipe. So, nice one John. There is no need to precook the rice as it will take on moisture from the squash.

SERVES 4

1 small handful of dried porcini mushrooms • 1 butternut
squash, halved and deseeded • olive oil • 1 red onion, peeled
and finely chopped • 1 clove of garlic, peeled and finely
chopped • 1 teaspoon coriander seeds, pounded • a pinch or
two of dried chilli, to taste • 2 sprigs of fresh rosemary, leaves
picked and finely chopped • 5 sun-dried tomatoes,
in oil, chopped • 100g basmati rice • ½ a handful
of pine nuts, lightly roasted

Soak the porcini in 140ml of boiling water for 5 minutes. Preheat the oven to 230°C/450°F/gas 8. Using a teaspoon, score and scoop out some extra flesh from the length of the squash (see pictures opposite). Finely chop this flesh with the squash seeds and place in a frying pan with 4 lugs of oil, the onion, garlic, coriander seeds, chilli, rosemary and sun-dried tomatoes. Fry for 4 minutes, or until softened. Add the porcini and half the soaking water. Cook for a further 2 minutes before seasoning with sea salt and black pepper. Stir in the rice and pine nuts, pack the mixture tightly into the 2 halves of the squash, then press together. Rub the skin of the squash with a little oil, wrap in tin foil, and bake in the oven for about 1 hour 15 minutes, or until soft and cooked through.

CALORIES	FAT	SAT FAT	PROTEIN	CARBS	SUGAR	SALT	FIBRE
308kcal	13.4g	1.8g	6.4g	43.4g	12.2g	0.8g	5.8g

Runner Beans with Tomato Sauce

SERVES 6

750g runner beans, sliced diagonally into 5cm pieces •
2 cloves of garlic, peeled and finely chopped • olive oil •
1 x 400g tin of quality plum tomatoes

Steam the beans in a foil-covered colander over a pot of boiling water, or blanch in boiling salted water until tender. While they're cooking, make a quick tomato sauce: fry the garlic in some oil, then add the tomatoes, breaking them up with a wooden spoon. Bring to the boil, then simmer for about 15 minutes, or until you have a thick sauce. Season to taste with sea salt and black pepper. When the beans are cooked, stir them into the sauce.

CALORIES	FAT	SAT FAT	PROTEIN	CARBS	SUGAR	SALT	FIBRE
64kcal	3.8g	0.6g	2.4g	5.7g	5.1g	0.2g	0.6g

THE WONDERFUL WORLD OF BREAD I'm still really mad about bread — I love it. It's so exciting. While me and my mate Bernie, who's a great baker, were trying to perfect our sourdough recipe it was hilarious 'cos we were like a couple of pregnant women on the phone each day seeing how our buns were proving. But that's what bread does to you. It's such a rewarding, therapeutic, tactile thing and you'll be so proud of yourself once you've cracked it.

And even though you can get all deep and cheffy about flours, fermentations and all that, I love that from one great simple bread recipe there's a million things you can do.

Anyone can make bread. I got kids to make the bread for the step-by-step photos, because if they can do it, then surely you can too. It's easy peasy. And just to prove to you that a little fantasy can stretch a bit of plain bread a long way, here's nine fantastic breads that will get you going on a Sunday morning. Roll your sleaves up and get stuck in.

Basic Bread Recipe

1kg strong bread flour, plus extra for dusting • 30g fresh yeast or 3 x 7g sachets of dried yeast • 2 tablespoons sugar

Stage 1: Making a Well

Pile the flour on to a clean surface and make a large well in the centre. Pour 300ml of tepid water into the well, then add the yeast, sugar and 1 level tablespoon of fine sea salt and stir with a fork.

Stage 2: Getting It Together

Slowly, but confidently, bring in the flour from the inside of the well. (You don't want to break the walls of the well, or the water will go everywhere.) Continue to bring the flour into the centre until you get a stodgy, porridgey consistency – then add another 300ml of tepid water. Continue to mix until it's stodgy again, then you can be more aggressive, bringing in all the flour, making the mix less sticky. Flour your hands and pat and push the dough together with all the remaining flour. (Certain flours need a little more or less water, so feel free to adjust.)

Stage 3: Kneading!

This is where you get stuck in. With a bit of elbow grease, simply push, fold, slap and roll the dough around, over and over, for 4 or 5 minutes until you have a silky and elastic dough.

Stage 4: First Prove

Flour the top of the dough. Put it into a bowl, cover with clingfilm, and allow it to prove for about half an hour, or until doubled in size – ideally in a warm, draught-free place. This will improve the flavour and texture of the dough and it's always exciting to know that the yeast has kicked into action.

Stage 5: Second Prove, Flavouring & Shaping

Once the dough has doubled in size, knock the air out for 30 seconds by bashing and squashing it. You can now shape it or flavour it as required – folded, filled, traybaked, whatever – and leave it to prove for a second time for 30 minutes to an hour, or until it has doubled in size once more. This is the most important part, as the second prove will give it the air that finally ends up being cooked into the bread, giving you the really light, soft texture that we all love in fresh bread. So remember – don't fiddle with it, just let it do its thing.

Stage 6: Cooking the Bread

Very gently place the bread dough on a flour-dusted baking tray and into a preheated oven. Don't slam the door or you'll lose the air that you need. Bake according to the time and temperature given with your chosen recipe. You can tell if it's cooked by tapping its bottom – if it sounds hollow it's done, if it doesn't then pop it back in for a little longer. Once cooked, place on a rack and allow it to cool for at least 30 minutes – fandabidozi. Feel free to freeze any leftover bread.

CALORIES	FAT	SAT FAT	PROTEIN	CARBS	SUGAR	SALT	FIBRE
141kcal	0.5g	0.1g	4.8g	31.1g	1.7g	0.4g	1.2g

THESE VALUES ARE BASED ON A 50G SLICE

Layered Focaccia with Cheese & Rocket

1 x Basic Bread Recipe (see page 236) • extra virgin olive oil •
170g Parmesan cheese, freshly grated • 200g Fontina, Cheddar
or good melting cheese, freshly grated • 140g mild Gorgonzola
cheese, crumbled • 2 large handfuls of rocket • ½ a bunch of
fresh marjoram, leaves picked • olive oil • optional: a few sprigs
of fresh sage or thyme

Follow the Basic Bread Recipe up to Stage 5 when you're shaping the dough. Roll it into a large rectangle around 1cm thick. Drape half of it into a medium to large flour-dusted baking tray, with half hanging over the side. On the half that is in the tray, drizzle over 3 good lugs of extra virgin olive oil, rub it into the dough, then add all the cheeses, the rocket, marjoram and a little sea salt and black pepper. Using your fingers, push it all into the dough. Fold the overhanging dough back on to the dough in the tray and then push around the edges so that you seal them together. What I do is tuck it under so it fits nicely into the tray. Rub the top with a little olive oil and rip over some fresh herbs like sage or thyme, if using.

Leave to prove and when doubled in size, bake in the oven at 180°C/350°F/gas 4 for 25 minutes, or until lightly golden and cooked through. Allow to sit for around 25 minutes before eating. This is a fantastic bread that can be cut into chunks, wrapped in greaseproof paper or tin foil and kept in the freezer to be reheated when you have midnight munchies.

CALORIES	FAT	SAT FAT	PROTEIN	CARBS	SUGAR	SALT	FIBRE
314kcal	10.8g	5.6g	14.4g	42.6g	2.8g	1.2g	1.8g

THESE VALUES ARE BASED ON A 50G SLICE

Gennaro Grande Cappella Rossa Calzone

My London 'father', Gennaro Contaldo, makes these delicious bites to use up all his leftover antipasti. They're great!

MAKES 8

1 onion, peeled and roughly chopped • 3 cloves of garlic, peeled and finely sliced • 1 aubergine, roughly chopped • olive oil • 3 courgettes, roughly chopped • 2 x 400g tins of quality plum tomatoes • optional: olives, stone in • 1 x Basic Bread Recipe (see page 236) • 1 bunch of fresh basil • 1 ball of buffalo mozzarella cheese

In a large pan, fry the onion, garlic and aubergine in a little oil on a high heat. After about 4 minutes, add the courgettes. Continue to fry for another 5 minutes, then add the tomatoes, breaking them up with a wooden spoon. Bring to the boil and simmer slowly for about 1 hour, or until quite thick and stodgy in texture – making sure it doesn't stick to the bottom. Remove from the heat, season well to taste with sea salt and black pepper, and add some olives, if using – just remove the stones first. Once cool, rip in the basil and mozzarella.

While it's cooking, make your dough and continue through the Basic Bread Recipe until Stage 5 where you divide the dough into 8 pieces. Roll into balls, using flour for dusting. Roll into little frisbee shapes just over ½cm thick. Place a good spoonful of the filling in the middle of each, brush the edges with a little water, then fold the rounds in half, pushing their edges to seal. Some people use a fork to do this but I just pinch them with my fingers. Dust with flour, do the same with all the others and move to a flour-dusted baking tray. Allow to sit for 5 minutes, then score the top of the bread to allow the filling to bubble over when cooking. Bake in the oven at 180°C/350°F/gas 4 for 20 minutes, or until golden and scrumptious-looking, and allow to cool. Always good for picnics or as portable food.

CALORIES	FAT	SAT FAT	PROTEIN	CARBS	SUGAR	SALT	FIBRE
540kcal	6.1g	2.6g	21.5g	106.5g	13.1g	1.4g	5.2g

SINCE 1916

Banana & Honey Bread

SERVES 10

6 ripe bananas • 1 x Basic Bread Recipe (see page 236) •
8 tablespoons runny honey • optional: 1 handful of almonds,
cracked or chopped

First of all, peel the bananas then purée in a blender – the mix will be surprisingly wet. Pour it into a measuring jug, then top up with water until you have 625ml. At Stage 1 of the Basic Bread Recipe, use this banana liquid instead of the water to flavour the bread and make it nice and chewy. Also add half the honey with the nuts, if using, to the dough at this point, then continue through the basic recipe.

At Stage 5 divide the dough into 10 balls. Pack these next to each other in a flour-dusted baking tin where they will prove together. Before putting into the oven drizzle generously with the rest of the honey so that the top of the bread will caramelize, going nice and golden. Bake in a preheated oven at 190°C/375°F/gas 5 for 20 minutes, or until golden. Allow to cool for a little while, but it's best served still warm with a little butter and a glass of milk for breakfast at the weekend while you read the paper. Also fantastic used in bread and butter pudding or simply heated up with a bit of ice cream.

CALORIES	FAT	SAT FAT	PROTEIN	CARBS	SUGAR	SALT	FIBRE
481kcal	3g	13.9g	13.9g	106.1g	30.6g	1g	3.8g

Walnut Bread

For this particular bread you need to use 500g wholemeal flour and 500g white flour instead of all white flour as used in the Basic Bread Recipe. Thought I'd better make that clear.

PS When using brown or wholemeal flours you often need to add a little more water to give you an elastic, pliable dough.

> 1 x Basic Bread Recipe (see page 236), using 500g wholemeal
> flour and 500g strong white flour • 450g shelled walnuts •
> 115g dried apricots, very finely chopped • 115g unsalted butter
> (at room temperature)

At Stage 1 of the Basic Bread Recipe remember to use both types of flour in place of just the white flour and continue to Stage 2.

Crush half the walnuts until coarse and the other half to a fine powder. At Stage 2 add these with the apricots and butter to the basic bread mix.

Carry on through the basic recipe until Stage 5. I normally divide this dough into 4, roll out into rolling-pin-shaped pieces and put these next to each other on a flour-dusted baking tray, but there's nothing stopping you cooking them in any shape. Allow the dough to double in size, then dust it with flour on the top. Bake in a preheated oven at 180°C/350°F/gas 4 for 30 minutes, or until lightly golden. Allow to cool for half an hour before using. Fantastic with cheese and pickle.

CALORIES	FAT	SAT FAT	PROTEIN	CARBS	SUGAR	SALT	FIBRE
394kcal	21.6g	4.8g	10.8g	41.6g	5.4g	0.5g	3.8g

THESE VALUES ARE BASED ON A 50G SLICE

Rolled Bread of Parma Ham, Nice Cheese, Egg & Basil

SERVES 12

1 x Basic Bread Recipe (see page 236) • 5 slices of Parma ham • 8 large eggs, boiled for 8 minutes and shelled • 200g mixed cheese, such as Cheddar, Fontina, Parmesan or any leftovers that need to be used up, grated • 1 bunch of fresh basil • optional: sun-dried tomatoes, in oil, or plum tomatoes and olives, stone in, halved • olive oil

Proceed through the Basic Bread Recipe until Stage 5, dusting the dough with flour as you shape it into a long rectangle about 1cm thick. This should end up being about 1 metre long and about 18 to 20cm wide.

Along the middle of the bread, lay out the Parma ham, eggs, cheese, basil and the tomatoes and olives (remove the stones first), if using. Drizzle with oil and season with a pinch of sea salt and black pepper. Pull the dough over the filling so it forms what looks like a cannelloni shape. Then what you need to do is bring one end round to the other so that they join up. Pinch and pat the two ends together firmly to form a doughnut-shaped loaf. Transfer to a flour-dusted baking tin, allow to prove for 15 minutes, then dust with flour. Bake in a preheated oven at 180°C/350°F/gas 4 for 35 minutes until golden. Allow to cool, then either transport to a picnic and carve it there – if you're lucky, it will still be a little warm in the middle – or eat there and then. Fantastic.

CALORIES	FAT	SAT FAT	PROTEIN	CARBS	SUGAR	SALT	FIBRE
439kcal	12.3g	5.2g	20.8g	65.5g	3.8g	1.7g	2.6g

Courgette Bread

1 x Basic Bread Recipe (see page 236) • 6 large courgettes,
grated • ½ a bunch of fresh thyme, leaves picked •
200g goat's cheese, crumbled

At Stage 1 of the Basic Bread Recipe, add 300ml of the water along with the courgettes and thyme. Mix around, using your hands to scrunch the bread together – you'll find that water will come out of the courgettes so you may not need to add the rest of the water at Stage 2, but add some if you feel the dough needs it. Carry on with the basic recipe up to Stage 5, until the dough is elastic and not sticky. Knead in the goat's cheese – it's an excellent combination. I normally shape the dough into a big round loaf and dust it with flour. Place on a flour-dusted baking tray and prove until doubled in size. Bake in a preheated oven at 180°C/350°F/gas 4 for around 30 minutes, or until crusty and hollow-sounding when tapped. It's superb toasted with cream cheese or used as sandwich bread.

CALORIES	FAT	SAT FAT	PROTEIN	CARBS	SUGAR	SALT	FIBRE
139kcal	2.2g	1.2g	6g	25g	2.4g	0.4g	1g

THESE VALUES ARE BASED ON A 50G SLICE

Onion Baguettes

MAKES 6

olive oil • 2 cloves of garlic, peeled and sliced •
½ a bunch of fresh thyme, leaves picked • 3 white onions,
peeled and finely sliced • 1 splash of white wine vinegar •
1 x Basic Bread Recipe (see page 236)

Into a pan, put 4 good lugs of oil, the sliced garlic and the thyme leaves. Add the onions, cover, and cook for 4 or 5 minutes. By then the moisture will have come out of the onions, so remove the lid and slowly cook away the liquid for a minute so you're left with nice, translucent, tasty onions – don't let them colour. Season to taste with sea salt and black pepper and add the vinegar.

While the onions are cooking, make the dough and continue through the Basic Bread Recipe until Stage 5, where you divide your dough into 6 pieces, dust with flour, and roll into classic baguette shapes. Move them to a flour-dusted baking tray, then rub the onion mixture over the top of each baguette. Allow to prove until doubled in size, then bake in a preheated oven at 180°C/350°F/gas 4 for 15 minutes, or until the bread is golden and crisp. The onions usually do burn a bit at the end, but that's all part of it – they end up being lovely. This is a fantastic sweet-tasting bread which is just nice, quite frankly, in a basket in the middle of the table before you tuck into dinner but is also pretty good with anything.

CALORIES	FAT	SAT FAT	PROTEIN	CARBS	SUGAR	SALT	FIBRE
344kcal	4.6g	0.7g	10.8g	69.3g	6.6g	0.9g	3.7g

THESE VALUES ARE BASED ON HALF A BAGUETTE

Sweet Cherry Focaccia Breakfast Stylie

1kg ripe cherries • 4 heaped tablespoons vanilla sugar •
1 x Basic Bread Recipe (see page 236) • 100g unsalted butter

Remove the pips from the cherries, either by simply pulling the pip out by hand or by using a cherry or olive pipper – this can be a bit mucky and might stain your shirt, so put a pinny on. Once you've disposed of all the pips, sprinkle 2 tablespoons of the vanilla sugar over the cherries and put to one side while you make the bread dough.

Work through the Basic Bread Recipe to Stage 5, when you're shaping the bread. You can divide the dough into two if you want to make 2 smaller ones. Push or roll out the dough to about 4cm thick. You can make them into rounds or fill a rectangular flour-dusted baking tray – it's up to you. Push the cherries into the dough – pushing your fingers right down to the bottom of the dough and sort of curling them under. Do this for about 2 minutes, then sprinkle the remaining sugar over the bread. Break the butter up into little knobs and put these on top. Leave to double in size, then place in the preheated oven at 180°C/350°F/gas 4 for 25 to 30 minutes, or until golden and cooked through. Best served warm with a little butter and a cup of milky coffee. It's also absolutely fantastic kept in chunks in the freezer, then reheated in the oven and served with vanilla ice cream. Yum yum.

CALORIES	FAT	SAT FAT	PROTEIN	CARBS	SUGAR	SALT	FIBRE
208kcal	4g	2.2g	5.5g	40.2g	10g	0.4g	1.2g

THESE VALUES ARE BASED ON A 50G SLICE

Sourdough Bread

Sourdough is the original, truly natural bread. We are talking biblical stuff here, because instead of using commercial yeast, we are making bread with natural yeasts from the air. Over the last year, my Aussie chef friend Bernie and I have been on a mission to bake the perfect sourdough bread and I think we've cracked it. Knotty and chewy with a holey texture and awesomely crisp crust, which keeps the moisture inside, sourdough is the ultimate loaf. The method stretches over a week – but once you've got your starter mix, you can make it every day.

It's worth knowing that you should use organic rye flour on the first day as it contains wild yeast and bacteria, and also that any additives or chemicals can stunt the growth of the microflora (a bit technical, but I thought you'd like to know!).

Monday Mix 500g of organic rye flour with enough water to make a soft dough, in a bowl. Put it outside for 1 hour, then place somewhere warm and cover with clingfilm.

Tuesday It will start to bubble. Leave it alone.

Wednesday The mix will continue to bubble and will go slightly grey. At this point, stir in a handful of flour and a little bit of water, enough to get the mixture back to the same consistency as on Monday. Leave it again, still covered.

Thursday Leave it alone.

Friday afternoon By now, you'll have a beery, malty-smelling, ashy-coloured mixture, full of natural yeasts, with loads of character. Make the bread by adding all of this starter dough mix to 1kg of strong flour, then adding enough water to make a firm, pliable dough that is not sticky. Knead it for a good 5 minutes. Remove a 500g piece of dough for your next starter before adding any sea salt, cover and put to one side, ready to repeat the process the next day, and so on, etc.

Add sea salt if you want to. Shape the dough and put it into a bowl or tin lined with a floured tea towel. Leave for 14 hours.

Saturday morning Bake the bread. Preheat the oven to 190°C/375°F/gas 5. Gently turn the dough out on to a floured baking tray, cut quite deep slashes into it, and bake for 1 hour, or until it is crisp and sounds hollow when tapped on the bottom. Allow to cool and enjoy fresh, or grilled as crostini. When it is stale, rip it up and add to soups.

CALORIES	FAT	SAT FAT	PROTEIN	CARBS	SUGAR	SALT	FIBRE
229kcal	0.8g	0.2g	6.8g	51.8g	0.4g	0.1g	4g

THESE VALUES ARE BASED ON A 50G SLICE

dess

DESSERTS A nice large dessert section this time as I've got a bit of a sweet tooth at the moment. I've included quite a few comforting recipes like Lovely Lemon Curdy Pud and Fruit Cobbler. All sorts of things to suit sweet-freaks.

I must tell you a really sweet story about one of my recipes from *The Naked Chef*. At the end of my fruit crumble recipe I had added, 'I bet you have loads of your own ideas – try them.' I recently had a letter from an old lady who said she had tried to be a bit imaginative but the results didn't taste very nice. It turned out that she had put some paprika crisps in the crumble mix. That really did make me laugh, but it's nice to think that there are some seriously adventurous birds out there!

Pukka Pineapple with Bashed-up Mint Sugar

As a child I always thought that a simple fruit option for dessert was flippin' boring and it never excited me in the slightest. But I now realize it was because no one did anything remotely exciting with the fruit. This recipe, however, I would definitely have enjoyed as a kid. It's one of those combinations that just explodes in your mouth and you can't get enough of it. Once you try it, you'll never forget it.

SERVES 4

1 ripe pineapple • optional: natural yoghurt, to serve •
2 tablespoons caster sugar • 1 bunch of fresh mint

Buy yourself a ripe pineapple – it should smell slightly sweet and you should be able to remove the leaves quite easily. Cut both ends off and peel the skin with a knife, removing any little black bits. Cut the pineapple into quarters and remove the slightly less tasty core, which I usually discard or suck on while preparing the rest of the dish. Finely slice the quarters, lengthways, as thin as you can. Lay out flat in one or two layers on a large plate. Don't refrigerate this – just put it to one side.

Take the plate to the table after dinner with a pot of yoghurt that can be passed round, then return with a pestle and mortar with the sugar in it. Your family or guests will probably think you've gone mad, especially if you ignore them while you do this, but pick the mint leaves and add them to the sugar. Bash the hell out of it in the pestle and mortar at the table. You'll see the sugar change colour and it will smell fantastic. It normally takes about 1 minute to do if you've got a good wrist action. Sprinkle the mint sugar over the plate of pineapple – making sure you don't let anyone nick any pineapple before you sprinkle the mint sugar over. What a fantastic thing. If you have any leftovers, you could always make a piña colada.

CALORIES	FAT	SAT FAT	PROTEIN	CARBS	SUGAR	SALT	FIBRE
82kcal	3g	0g	0.6g	20.6g	20.5g	0g	1.5g

Cannoli Siciliana

This is a great little dessert that my mate Gennaro Contaldo, the Italian stallion, taught me to make. Cannoli biscuits are filled with lovely sweet ricotta and can be flavoured with absolutely anything. They can even be dipped into melted chocolate. You can buy them pre-made from all good Italian delis and most good supermarkets (if they haven't got them then tell them to order them in). They're basically deep-fried, sweetened pasta biscuits which are really light and crispy.

MAKES 12

2 large punnets of raspberries • 6 heaped tablespoons vanilla sugar • 200g ricotta cheese (buffalo is best) • 100g quality dark chocolate (70%), chopped • 50g shelled pistachios, chopped • 50g glacé fruit, chopped • 12 cannoli biscuits • icing sugar

I love to make a raspberry sauce to go with these cannoli biscuits – just throw the raspberries into a small pan with 3 tablespoons of the sugar, bring to the boil, simmer for 1 minute then allow to cool.

Meanwhile, put the ricotta and the remaining 3 tablespoons of sugar into a food processor and blitz for 1 minute, or until shiny and smooth. If you taste the ricotta now it should be beautifully sweet. Some ricottas need more sugar than others, so taste and adjust to your preference. Scoop it out into a bowl and add the chocolate, pistachios and glacé fruit. Feel free to improvise with flavours here – you can only learn by trying. Put the mixture into a piping bag and pipe all the way through your cannoli biscuits. You can cut a small corner off a plastic or sandwich bag if you haven't got a piping bag. Place 3 biscuits on each plate, drizzled with your raspberry sauce and sprinkled with a little icing sugar. Lovely.

CALORIES	FAT	SAT FAT	PROTEIN	CARBS	SUGAR	SALT	FIBRE
252kcal	12.7g	4.1g	4.6g	33.1g	19.7g	0.1g	1.1g

Yoghurt with Blueberry Jam & Elderflower Cordial

This is a fantastic quick recipe for those days when you don't want to spend ages knocking up a dessert. Or it can be a really good intermediate palate cleanser before your main course. It can be made with any jam you like, but blueberry jam is particularly tasty. Try strawberry or raspberry, too.

SERVES 4

500g Greek or natural yoghurt • 4 tablespoons blueberry
jam • 8 tablespoons elderflower cordial • 4 sprigs of fresh mint

Divide the yoghurt between 4 dessert bowls or small glasses. Spoon over the blueberry jam, cover with the elderflower cordial, and top with a sprig of mint.

CALORIES	FAT	SAT FAT	PROTEIN	CARBS	SUGAR	SALT	FIBRE
235kcal	11.9g	7.4g	5.8g	26.2g	22.9g	0.3g	0.5g

Fruit Cobbler

This is a fantastic American recipe equivalent to our crumble. It's particularly good with strawberries and rhubarb, but you can use any fruit combo you like; about 700g of fruit in total should do it.

SERVES 6

FRUIT

2 apricots, stoned and sliced • 1 pear, cored and thickly sliced • 1 punnet of blackberries • 1 punnet of blueberries • 1 punnet of raspberries • ½ an eating apple, grated • 5 tablespoons sugar • balsamic vinegar

TOPPING

170g unsalted butter (cold) • 225g self-raising flour • 70g sugar, plus extra for sprinkling • 130ml buttermilk

Preheat the oven to 190°C/375°F/gas 5. Put the fruit into a pan with the sugar and a good lug of balsamic vinegar, place the pan over the heat, and cook gently until the juices begin to run from the berries. Pour into an ovenproof dish.

Meanwhile, make the topping. Rub the butter into the flour until the mixture resembles fine breadcrumbs. Add the sugar and a pinch of sea salt, stir well, then add the buttermilk to form a loose scone-type mixture. Spoon this over the hot fruit (to get a cobbled effect, flick balls of dough randomly over the fruit), sprinkle with a little caster sugar, and bake in the oven for 30 minutes, or until golden brown. Tasty served with vanilla ice cream.

CALORIES	FAT	SAT FAT	PROTEIN	CARBS	SUGAR	SALT	FIBRE
496kcal	24.2g	15g	5.7g	67.8g	38.2g	0.5g	2.7g

Chocolate Cambridge Cream

Cambridge cream is basically a very similar recipe to crème brûlée.

3 vanilla pods • 200ml milk • 350ml double cream • 8 large
egg yolks • 70g caster sugar, plus extra for sprinkling •
1 heaped teaspoon quality cocoa powder • 100g good dark
chocolate (70%), bashed up finely

Run a knife along the length of the vanilla pods, scraping out the seeds, then chop up the pods. Put the seeds and pods into a thick-bottomed pan with the milk and cream. Simmer slowly for 5 minutes for the flavour to infuse. In a bowl that will sit on top of your pan, whisk the egg yolks, sugar and cocoa powder for 1 minute. Still slowly whisking, add the vanilla-flavoured milk and cream and keep whisking until well mixed. Add 2.5cm of hot water to the dirty pan, bring to a simmer, and put the bowl on top of the pan. Cook the custard slowly over the simmering water for 5 minutes, or until it coats the back of a spoon, stirring often. Get a jug, then push the custard through a fine sieve into it. Discard the vanilla pods.

Preheat the oven to 150°C/300°F/gas 2. Put 8 small ovenproof ramekins into a high-sided roasting tray. Divide the chocolate between them and shake flat. Carefully divide the custard mix between the dishes, making sure the chocolate isn't disturbed. Fill the tray with water until it is about halfway up the sides of your dishes. Cook in the oven for 20 minutes, or until slightly wobbly in the middle. Keep your eyes peeled and don't let the custards cook solid – remember that all ovens cook differently. Allow to cool (you can refrigerate these for up to 3 days if you like, but I like it best on the night at room temperature), then sprinkle with some sugar and caramelize with one of those small blowtorches (or you can boil 6 tablespoons of sugar with a couple of tablespoons of water until you have golden caramel and carefully pour this over the top if you're stuck).

CALORIES	FAT	SAT FAT	PROTEIN	CARBS	SUGAR	SALT	FIBRE
427kcal	36.6g	20g	6.6g	18.1g	17.4g	0.1g	1.5g

Sesame Seed Toffee Snaps

These are great served with the lovely chocolate mousse on page 278. Caramel can cause quite bad burns, so be careful and keep your eyes peeled – don't get the kids involved in cooking this one.

MAKES 24

450g caster sugar • 200g pack of sesame seeds

Put the sugar and 8 to 10 tablespoons of water into a pan on a medium heat. Use a spoon to stir together – it will become a syrup. Carry on cooking until light golden (but don't stir too much at this stage or sugar crystals will form in the syrup and you don't want this to happen), then add the sesame seeds and continue to cook until dark golden. Pour out the sesame seed caramel on to an oiled non-stick tray. Use a palette knife to push it out to about ½cm thick (even thinner if you can). Allow to cool for about 15 minutes and you will have one big sesame seed caramel biscuit. Bash it up into small pieces.

CALORIES	FAT	SAT FAT	PROTEIN	CARBS	SUGAR	SALT	FIBRE
124kcal	4.9g	0.9g	1.6g	19.8g	19.7g	0g	1g

Cheeky Chocolate Mousse

SERVES 10

225g quality dark chocolate (70%), bashed up • 40g unsalted
butter, cut into pieces • 350ml double cream • 2 large eggs •
2 tablespoons runny honey • 1 tablespoon Amaretto

In a bowl over some gently simmering water, slowly melt the chocolate and butter together, then remove from the heat. In a separate bowl, semi-whip the cream (until soft peaks; not too stiff). In a third bowl, whisk the eggs and honey until light and fluffy, then fold in the Amaretto, melted chocolate mixture and cream – gently, so you don't lose too much air. Pour into some small glasses and leave to chill for at least 1 hour. Delicious served with Sesame Seed Toffee Snaps (see page 275).

CALORIES	FAT	SAT FAT	PROTEIN	CARBS	SUGAR	SALT	FIBRE
364kcal	32.5g	19.7g	4.1g	11.9g	10.8g	0.1g	2.7g

Chocolate & Whole Orange Pudding

A pudding with a lovely surprise in the centre when you cut it open. The orange peel is cooked like marmalade and its sharpness goes well with the sweet chocolate.

SERVES 8

85g unsalted butter, plus extra for greasing • 50g quality dark chocolate (70%) • 170g self-raising flour • 50g quality cocoa powder • 170g caster sugar • 2 large eggs •
2 tablespoons milk

FILLING

1 orange – preferably a thin-skinned navel variety •
85g unsalted butter • 85g caster sugar

Bring some water to the boil in a pan (in which you're going to steam the pudding later), and put in the whole orange to boil fast for 10 minutes with the lid on.

Meanwhile, grease a 1.2 litre pudding basin. Melt the butter with the chocolate in a bowl set over a pan of hot water. Put the flour and cocoa into a mixing bowl; add the melted butter and chocolate, then the sugar, eggs and milk, and mix well. Put about two-thirds of the mixture into the basin, making a well in the middle.

By this time the orange should have been boiling for about 10 minutes, and the peel should be nice and soft. Remove it carefully from the water. Prick the orange all over with a fork or skewer and place it in the middle of the pudding mix. You can (with care, as it's still hot) cut the orange into segments, if you want to check for pips or cut off the stringy bits of orange in the middle, then put it back together again (it does make it easier for serving), although I don't usually bother.

Dice the butter and dot it round the orange with the sugar, then cover with the remaining pudding mixture. Cover the pudding with greaseproof paper, then with tin foil, and place in the pan of boiling water (it should come halfway up the sides of the basin). Steam for 2 hours. Don't forget to check now and then to see if the water needs topping up.

Turn the pudding out on to a serving dish and serve with custard or cream.

CALORIES	FAT	SAT FAT	PROTEIN	CARBS	SUGAR	SALT	FIBRE
443kcal	23.2g	13.9g	5.9g	55.8g	37.9g	0.3g	1.9g

King of Puddings

SERVES 6

4 large eggs • 550ml milk • 100g fine breadcrumbs •
225g sugar (preferably vanilla sugar) • 4 level tablespoons jam
(raspberry is really nice)

Preheat the oven to 150ºC/300ºF/gas 2. Separate 3 of the eggs. Put the yolks into a bowl with the remaining whole egg and beat together. Add the milk, breadcrumbs and 85g of the sugar. Put the jam on the bottom of a pie dish and spread it evenly. Pour the custardy egg and milk mixture over the jam. Bake in the oven for 1 hour, or until set.

Whisk the remaining 3 egg whites until stiff, then slowly add the remaining sugar until it is all mixed in. Pile it on top of the custard, then bake in the oven for a further 15 to 20 minutes, or until the meringue is set and lightly browned.

CALORIES	FAT	SAT FAT	PROTEIN	CARBS	SUGAR	SALT	FIBRE
356kcal	6.4g	2.3g	9.7g	67.3g	54.1g	0.4g	1.1g

Lovely Lemon Curdy Pud

This is really tasty and dead easy to make – my sister Anna loves it! It looks good cooked in a clear dish, as it goes into layers as it cooks, with a sort of lemon curdy custard at the bottom and a spongy meringuey top. Mmmmmmm . . . very delicious!

SERVES 4

1 lemon • 55g unsalted butter, plus extra for greasing •
115g sugar (vanilla sugar is nice) • 2 large eggs, separated •
55g self-raising flour • 285ml milk

Preheat the oven to 200°C/400°F/gas 6. Finely grate the lemon zest into a mixing bowl, then add the butter and sugar and cream together. Add the egg yolks and flour and beat in, then add the milk and 3 tablespoons of lemon juice and mix well.

Whisk the egg whites in a separate bowl until stiff, then add the rest of the mixture. Mix it all well but don't over-mix it; you don't want the air to come out of the egg whites. Pour into a greased ovenproof dish, stand the dish in a roasting tin about a third full of water, then bake in the oven for 45 minutes, or until the top is set and spongy and it's a nice golden colour.

CALORIES	FAT	SAT FAT	PROTEIN	CARBS	SUGAR	SALT	FIBRE
334kcal	15.3g	8.7g	7.5g	44.7g	33.8g	0.3g	0.7g

Summer Fruit, Elderflower & Prosecco Jelly

This is a great dessert that is really tasty. It freshens the palate and you can make it before you need it – it keeps for about 3 days. You can make one large jelly in a tureen mould or dish, or you can do individual ones. Use any combination of fruit, but not pineapple or kiwi fruit, as the jelly won't set if you do.

SERVES 10

8 punnets of mixed soft fruit, such as blackberries, raspberries, strawberries, blueberries • 4 leaves of gelatine • 140ml elderflower cordial • 2 heaped tablespoons caster sugar • 420ml prosecco, chilled

First of all, decide whether you want to make one big jelly or small individual ones. If you are making a big one, it's a good idea to line it with clingfilm. Put the ripe fruit into the mould or moulds and refrigerate. Put the gelatine leaves into a bowl with a little cold water to soak for a minute, then drain and add the gelatine back to the bowl, along with the cordial. Rest above a pan of water over a medium heat and stir constantly until the gelatine and cordial become a syrup. At this point you can add the sugar, stir till dissolved, then remove the bowl from the heat and let it sit at room temperature for a minute or so.

Take the fruit and prosecco out of the fridge. The idea is that the fruit, moulds and prosecco are all chilled, so the bubbles stay in the jelly when it sets and they fizz in your mouth when you eat it – beautiful! Pour the prosecco into the cordial mix, then pour this over the fruit. Some of the fruit might rise to the top, so using your finger, just push the fruit down into the jelly mix so that it is sealed and will then keep well in the fridge. Put back into the fridge for 1 hour, or until set.

To serve, dip the mould into a bowl of hot water to loosen the outside of the jelly, then turn it out on to a plate. Great served with a little crème fraîche.

CALORIES	FAT	SAT FAT	PROTEIN	CARBS	SUGAR	SALT	FIBRE
169kcal	0.7g	0.1g	3.7g	31.5g	27.9g	0g	7.3g

What a great tart – chewy, with a gorgeous combo of pine nuts and honey. It was introduced to me by one of my good mates, Jethro, who's my pastry chef at Monte's. I met him in Australia and he's always been good with tarts! Thanks, Jethro. 'You is the man.'

Jethro Tart

250g pine nuts • 250g unsalted butter • 250g caster sugar •
3 large eggs • 4 tablespoons Greek fig tree honey, or any runny
honey • 115g plain flour

PASTRY

100g unsalted butter • 100g icing sugar • 225g plain flour •
2 large egg yolks • 2 tablespoons cold milk

You can make the pastry by hand or in a food processor. Cream the butter, sugar and a pinch of sea salt together, then rub or pulse in the flour and egg yolks. When the mixture looks like coarse breadcrumbs, add the milk. Gently pat together to form a small ball of dough. Wrap and leave to rest for 1 hour.

Carefully cut thin slices of the pastry (or you can roll out if you prefer) and place in and around the bottom and sides of a 30cm tart tin. Push the pastry together and level out and tidy up the sides. Cover and leave to rest in the freezer for 1 hour. Preheat the oven to 180°C/350°F/gas 4, and bake the pastry for 15 minutes, or until lightly golden. Reduce the oven temperature to 170°C/325°F/gas 3.

While the pastry is in the oven, toast the pine nuts under the grill. If you're like me you'll forget about them and they'll burn, so keep your eyes peeled – they don't take long to colour. Using a spatula, or a food processor, whip the butter and sugar until light and fluffy. Stir in the pine nuts, add the eggs one at a time, then fold in the honey, flour and a pinch of sea salt. Spoon into the tart shell and bake for 30 to 35 minutes, or until beautifully golden.

Great served with grilled figs, crème fraîche and a little lemon thyme.

CALORIES	FAT	SAT FAT	PROTEIN	CARBS	SUGAR	SALT	FIBRE
539kcal	35.3g	14.6g	7g	51.7g	32g	0.2g	1g

Pannacotta with Roasted Rhubarb

SERVES 4

200ml whole milk • 2 vanilla pods, halved lengthways and seeds
removed • 200ml double cream • 1 lemon • 1½ leaves of
gelatine, soaked in water • 70g icing sugar • 200g rhubarb •
2 tablespoons caster sugar • 5cm piece of ginger, peeled
and grated • 1 x 2.5cm cinnamon stick • 100ml Champagne,
prosecco or other sparkling wine

Put the milk, vanilla pods and seeds, and half the cream into a small pan. Finely grate in the lemon zest and slowly simmer for 10 minutes, or until reduced by a third. Remove from the heat and stir in the soaked gelatine leaves until dissolved. Allow to cool a little, then place in the fridge, stirring occasionally until the mixture coats the back of a spoon. Remove the vanilla pods.

Whip the icing sugar and remaining cream together. Mix the two cream mixtures together. Divide into 4 serving moulds (I use little moulds, espresso cups or small glasses). Cover and chill for at least an hour.

Meanwhile chop the rhubarb into 4cm pieces, sprinkle with the caster sugar and grill until lightly browned. Gently heat the ginger, cinnamon and Champagne together, then pour over the roasted rhubarb, cover, and leave for about 30 minutes for the flavours to do their bit.

To serve, sometimes I'll dip the mould or cup into some simmering water to loosen the pannacotta a little, then turn it out on to a plate next to some rhubarb with its juice (remove the cinnamon). Or you can just put the rhubarb on top of the cups or glasses of pannacotta and serve from there. Both ways are cool. Also gorgeous served with fresh figs and honey or caramelized blood oranges.

PS Nice scattered with a few fresh baby basil leaves.

CALORIES	FAT	SAT FAT	PROTEIN	CARBS	SUGAR	SALT	FIBRE
397kcal	27.8g	17.2g	3.3g	30.4g	30.1g	0.1g	0.7g

BEVVY BEVOIRES I'm still very partial to a good old drink. And it's nice to know that you lot are, too. My lord, how people went mad for the vodka watermelon from *Return of the Naked Chef* – from teenagers to OAPs I wasn't sure who was worse. I even caught my mate Jimmy injecting passion fruit and grapes with vodka – what a nutter! You can tell he's a student. But if you want something to swear by this time, have a go at a Sidecar, which is my biggest luxury at the moment. Great for calming you down and kickstarting the night. Just to show that I'm not obsessed with cocktails, I've included some absolutely amazing soft drinks, including Christmas in a Glass, which is pure joy. It's mandarin juice with a little mint; my family drinks it on Christmas Day. And there's a recipe for ginger beer, which is the most refreshing thing on a hot summer day. Have a look and have a drink on me.

The Best Hot Chocolate

This is a great way to make the best hot chocolate, cappuccino or frothy milk without having to buy expensive machinery. All you need is a good-sized thermos flask or a plastic jug with a screw-top lid. I've even made pukka Ovaltine like this!

SERVES 2

500ml milk • 2 tablespoons quality drinking chocolate •
optional: sugar, to taste • 1 handful of marshmallows

This takes around 3 or 4 minutes to make. First put the milk into a pan. Bring to a simmer – not a boil – and while it's heating, put 1 tablespoon of choccie powder and sugar (if using) to taste into each mug. Add a little warmish milk from the pan to each mug – you just need enough to dissolve the chocolate powder. At this point, plonk a few marshmallows into each mug. When the milk is at a simmer, carefully pour it into a plastic jug or flask. I normally do this over a sink as I always end up spilling a bit (the trick is to have a big enough jug or flask so the milk only half fills it – you need the extra space for shaking and frothing).

Screw the lid on tightly, place a cloth over the lid for safety, and shake hard for 1 minute. Remove the lid, minding the steam, and pour the milk into your mugs. A little stir and you can slurp your way to heaven!

CALORIES	FAT	SAT FAT	PROTEIN	CARBS	SUGAR	SALT	FIBRE
173kcal	5.2g	3.3g	10.5g	23g	8.3g	0.4g	0g

Easy Peasy Ginger Beer

Ginger beer is one of my favourite things in the world, especially blooming good in the summer when it's getting hot. I can't think of anything more sexy than having a big jug of iced ginger beer on the table with a barbecue on a hot day. The classic real ginger beers use a starter, and these are fantastic but slow, so here's my shortcut for getting amazing results taking hardly any time.

SERVES 4

140g ginger • 4 tablespoons muscovado sugar • 3 lemons •
1 litre soda water or sparkling mineral water •
a few sprigs of fresh mint

First of all you need to grate the ginger on a coarse cheese grater – you can leave the skin on if you like. Put the ginger with its pulpy juice into a bowl and sprinkle in the muscovado sugar. Remove the rind from 2 of the lemons in strips with a speed-peeler, add to the bowl and slightly bash and squash with something heavy like a pestle or a rolling pin. Just do this for 10 seconds, to mix up all the flavours. Squeeze the juice from all 3 lemons and add most of it to the bowl. Pour in the soda or sparkling water. Allow to sit for 10 minutes, then taste. You may feel that the lemons are slightly too sour, therefore add a little more sugar; if it's slightly too sweet, add a little more lemon juice. To be honest, these amounts are always a little variable so just follow your own taste. Pass the ginger beer through a coarse sieve into a large jug and add lots of ice and some sprigs of mint.

CALORIES	FAT	SAT FAT	PROTEIN	CARBS	SUGAR	SALT	FIBRE
74kcal	0.3g	0.1g	0.8g	19.0g	6.6g	0.2g	0g

Christmas in a Glass

Last Christmas we had so many tangerines and mandarins in the house, we knew that they were all going to go mouldy and dodgy. So we kept a few, then cut the rest in half and juiced them. Then we put the juice through a coarse sieve to remove any chunky pith and added a few mint leaves. We served this chilled on Christmas morning and it was an absolute joy. All we could say was that it was Christmas in a glass. Every time we took a sip it tasted like Christmas, if you can imagine what Christmas tastes like. But seriously, this is one of the best drinks that I've ever had. When mandarins, tangerines or clementines are in season and cheap, it's a great drink to use with maybe champagne, prosecco, in cocktails or just as juice on its own. Give it a try. You will need about 5 mandarins per person.

CALORIES	FAT	SAT FAT	PROTEIN	CARBS	SUGAR	SALT	FIBRE
51kcal	0g	0g	1g	12.3g	12.2g	0.1g	0g

Mango Lassi

This Indian drink is like a mango milkshake and is delicious.

SERVES 4

250g natural yoghurt • 130ml milk • 130ml canned mango pulp
or 200g fresh mango, stone removed and sliced •
optional: sugar, to taste

Put all the ingredients into a blender and blend for 2 minutes, then pour into individual glasses and serve. The lassi can be kept refrigerated for up to 24 hours.

CALORIES	FAT	SAT FAT	PROTEIN	CARBS	SUGAR	SALT	FIBRE
95kcal	3.3g	2.1g	4.4g	12.6g	12.5g	0.1g	0g

Sidecar

This is a superb little cocktail and the recipe is from Tony Debok at a bar called Daddy-O in New York. Definitely one to try.

MAKES 2 SMALL OR 1 LARGE

2 tablespoons caster sugar, plus extra to serve •
50ml good brandy • 25ml Cointreau • 2–3 fresh limes

First stir the sugar and 3 tablespoons of boiling water together until dissolved, then add the brandy, Cointreau and lime juice. Add some ice and shake well. Taste a little – you may want to add some more lime to give it an edge. Serve up in a martini glass with a sugar rim and a twist of lime zest.

CALORIES	FAT	SAT FAT	PROTEIN	CARBS	SUGAR	SALT	FIBRE
179kcal	0g	0g	0.1g	25.2g	25.2g	0g	0g

Margarita

SERVES 1

1 lime • 50ml tequila • 25ml Cointreau

Cut a wedge from the lime and put to one side. Squeeze 25ml of lime juice into a shaker, then add the other ingredients. Shake well and serve in a martini glass with a salt rim and the lime wedge.

CALORIES	FAT	SAT FAT	PROTEIN	CARBS	SUGAR	SALT	FIBRE
238kcal	0g	0g	0.1g	18.7g	18.7g	1g	0g

Jum & Bender

This great little cocktail was made by the barman after me and my mate Ben started working at Monte's.

SERVES 1

3 passion fruit • a little Champagne to top up
• a dash of grenadine

Halve the passion fruit and push the juice through a coarse sieve to separate the lovely flavour from the seeds. Discard the seeds but keep all the pulpy juice which will have gathered on the underside of the sieve. Pour into a tall glass and top up with Champagne and a dash of grenadine. Cheers!

AND FINALLY ...
YOU ARE WHAT YOU EAT

I recently met a fantastic lady called Jane Clarke who is a dietitian in Soho. In actual fact, she hates the word dietitian so she calls herself a 'food-loving nutritionist'. The thing I love about Jane is that she enjoys cooking with all kinds of flavours and she believes that a good diet isn't just about losing weight. If we eat well it will help us to feel livelier and more healthy, and can make us look better and even perform better at work. While I was chatting to Jane, she suggested a few things that we can all do in order to ensure that we have a better diet. It's common-sense stuff that we can all benefit from, so check it out and have a go at some of these things.

• *Drink more water* It's good to have 2.5 litres a day. Water is great for fending off headaches, easing digestion, improving your skin and will give you more energy. It also helps to release all the vitamins and minerals from your food into your body. There's nothing wrong with drinking tap water – if you don't like the taste then get yourself a filter.

• *Eat slowly and enjoy your food* If you eat your food too quickly your brain won't pick up on the fact that you're actually full up as quickly as it should, so you will carry on stuffing yourself until you've eaten too much.

• *Eat 'real' food rather than low-calorie food* This may surprise you, but a little bit of 'real' full-fat food can be better for you than many of the low-fat versions. Be sure to check food labels so you understand exactly what it is that you are buying. To keep your heart healthy, use olive or vegetable oils rather than over-relying on butter.

• *Eat small meals often* Don't skip breakfast and stuff yourself at lunchtime or your food will sit heavily and overload your stomach.

• *Celebrate good carbs* Starchy carbs are a wonderful thing – they make us feel happy, satisfied and energetic, and provide us with a large proportion of the energy we need to function. Choose fibre-rich wholegrain and wholewheat varieties when you can, which take longer to break down, are slow-releasing, and give us a more sustained level of energy, also helping us feel fuller for longer.

• *Resist alcohol on an empty stomach* This is a tip which I completely agree with (as I have done this and suffered the consequences!). It will send your energy levels crashing and you'll feel shattered as your blood sugar level is lower. You'll feel that you've got to eat something immediately – whether it be crisps, a doner kebab or a curry. A carb-based meal before you start drinking can help slow the absorption of alcohol, and having a glass of water in between alcoholic drinks can also help to prevent dehydration, reducing the likelihood of a bad hangover.

It's much better to eat and drink at the same time which means you can still get tiddly but without all the negative effects on your digestive system. If you haven't got time, then a glass of milk or a banana before you start drinking should stop the alcohol having such a drastic effect.

• *Watch the caffeine* Things like coffee, tea and cola all contain caffeine. If you have too much the caffeine produces adrenaline which will stress you out more. Stick to 2 cups of good coffee, and then maybe drink herbal tea or hot water with a slice of ginger or lemon, which should help you feel calmer and sleep better.

• *Eat more protein* We all eat enough protein, but not many of us are eating enough fish (especially the oily fish), eggs, seafood, lean meat, pulses, nuts, grains, which are better for us than processed meats. Protein is the building blocks of our bodies. It is essential for the growth and repair of muscles, as well as building hormones, enzymes and the antibodies in our immune system.

• *It's really worth eating lots of fruit and veg* Hopefully everyone knows that eating at least 5 portions of veg and fruit a day can help to prevent things like heart disease and cancer – find the ones you like, and work them into your diet. Fruit and veg come in so many shapes, sizes, colours, flavours and textures, so eat as wide a variety as possible to get a variety of vitamins and minerals.

Recipes marked v are suitable for vegetarians
Page numbers in bold indicate photography

A

NICE ONE GUYS I'd just like to say a special thanks to all the people who help me do what I do – all of whom are now great friends of mine. I'll start with my family ... My amazing wife Jools for marrying me and putting up with me, to my gorgeous mum and dad as always for everything, to the rest of the Oliver, Palmer and Norton families for their support, especially that Mrs Qwwyyzzy Norton • David Loftus, the most talented and patient photographer I've ever known, a best mate and great travelling partner. Bring on the Sidecars bro! PS Much love to Debbie, Paros and Pascale • Thanks to my fantastic assistants Louise Holland, Nicola Duguid and Lisa Norton for your true dedication and friendship xxx • Thanks to my best friends for being my best friends: Andy the gasman, he's still single and available, Jimmy Doherty the nature boy, Dan Brightman the Cornish Surfer, and all the other nutters I grew up with, Willy Wilson, Gray Boy, Ruby Quince and the rest • To Gennaro and Liz and all of the Passione team in Charlotte Street for being like a second family xxx • All my love to my beloved Lindsey Jordan, my editor. And to Tom Weldon, my publisher, who has been surprisingly calm through the whole book! Thanks ... what can I say? To Johnny Boy Hamilton for putting up with me being so intense over the design and look of the book, and for working around my mad life on Sundays and late nights I should thank your wife – really sorry, Claire. Massive respect to Jo Seaton, Annie Lee, Nicky Barneby, James Holland, Sophie Brewer, Tora Orde-Powlett, Keith Taylor, John Bond and Miss Moneypenny, Harrie 'he's free and available' Evans, Peter Bowron and all the brilliant Penguin sales team • Patricia Llewellyn, my TV producer and the infamous voice behind *The Naked Chef* you are the best. Thanks for everything, Niall and Ewen, the directors of the programmes, and to the rest of the team – Peter Gillbe, Nina, Lucy, Rowan, Chris, Patrick, Jon, Louise, Luke Cardiff and Richard Hill • Mark Gray, Paul Hunt,

Khoi, Josh and Tessa for all their work on jamieoliver.com • To the lovely Ginny Rolfe, wonder woman, and her fella John the baker • Kate Habershom • Harriet Docker • Richard at the Warehouse • Cheers to my agents, Borra, Aden, Michelle and Martine from Deborah McKenna Ltd • Lance Reynolds • Sheila Keating, for being an absolute diamond • To lovely Lincoln, Jane and all the kids, Sunny, Jake and Honey, bless • Jane Clarke • To Uncle Geoff, Heather, Ashley and Stephanie • To my mate Bender the Aussie and all my chefs and managers at Monte's • To Mr Frost, the one who made me famous • To the mad liver lips Charlie, and to Maria for sorting me out big time • Thanks to Das and all the team from Rasa in London for their support and genius Indian food • And, last but not least, a massive thanks to my suppliers: To Patricia from La Fromagerie, the best cheese shop in the world • David Gleave from Liberty Wines for helping me source some fantastic olive oils and wines from Italy • Jekka, the loveliest organic herb lady in the world. Get your window boxes done, jekkasherbfarm. com • Birgit Erath at the Spice Shop (www.thespiceshop.co.uk) • Everyone at Borough Market in London for their amazing Fridays and Saturdays – such passion and hard work; you make my weekends exciting. Here's to more markets like yours • To the best fishmongers … George at Golborne Fisheries, Ben at Rossmore Fisheries, The Southbank Seafood Company Ltd and John at Blagdens for his great game • The butchers: Kevin at Allen's, Brian at Randalls and Gary at M. Moen & Sons • Rushton, Greg and all the boys at George Allens Vegetables for all the early calls • Hyams and Cockerton for all the fruit and veg • To Sir Peter Davis and the Sainsbury's posse for letting me launch exciting projects like the herb range and here's to more in the future.

Sorted . . . I'm off